DISMISSED

DISMISSED

Tackling the Biases That Undermine Our Health Care

ANGELA MARSHALL, MD

WITH **KATHY PALOKOFF**

CITADEL PRESS
Kensington Publishing Corp.
www.kensingtonbooks.com

This book is dedicated to my children, husband,
patients, and the next generation.
May they live in a world where they are never dismissed.

—A. M.

CITADEL PRESS BOOKS are published by

Kensington Publishing Corp.
119 West 40th Street
New York, NY 10018

Copyright © 2023 Marshall Health Enterprises, LLC

PUBLISHER'S NOTE
This book is sold to readers with the understanding that while the publisher aims to inform, enlighten, and provide accurate general information regarding the subject matter covered, the publisher is not engaged in providing medical, psychological, financial, legal, or other professional services. If the reader needs or wants professional advice or assistance, the services of an appropriate professional should be sought. Case studies featured in this book are composites based on the author's years of practice and do not reflect the experiences of any individual person.

All Kensington titles, imprints, and distributed lines are available at special quantity discounts for bulk purchases for sales promotions, premiums, fund-raising, educational, or institutional use. Special book excerpts or customized printings can also be created to fit specific needs. For details, write or phone the office of the Kensington sales manager: Kensington Publishing Corp., 119 West 40th Street, New York, NY 10018, attn: Sales Department; phone 1-800-221-2647.

CITADEL PRESS and the Citadel logo are Reg. U.S. Pat. & TM Off.

ISBN: 978-0-8065-4204-1

First Citadel hardcover printing: April 2023

10 9 8 7 6 5 4 3 2 1

Printed in the United States of America

Library of Congress Control Number: 2022948696

ISBN: 978-0-8065-4206-5 (e-book)

Contents

Introduction

As a primary care doctor who has seen more than fifty thousand patients in the last twenty years, I have a different perspective on health care than many other providers. Only 2 percent of primary care doctors in the United States are Black women, and just a handful of practices specialize in women's health. My own experiences growing up in poverty also gave me a lot of life lessons about prejudice, racism, and classism.

Over the past few years, I have taken visible public leadership roles in women's health, particularly for Black women, to raise my voice as an advocate, change maker, and educator. As I moved beyond my own personal experiences and geography, I began hearing stories of fear and mistrust of the medical system by all sorts of patients, not only Black women. Explicit and implicit bias were everyday encounters for people outside of the racial, economic, and physical norm. Many people found their doctors' offices to be judgmental places where they did not feel safe or respected.

Then COVID began its course of devastation, and Black Lives Matter entered mainstream America. Disparities in our health-care system became painfully obvious with the disproportionate number of deaths among African Americans, Native Americans, and Hispanic Americans. My co-writer, Kathy, and I began conversations about varieties of bias in health care. She is a writer and White woman whose family experienced prejudice and death because of being Jewish. She is also "fat" (her description) and "old" (again, her description), two more targets for bias in health care. We realized that bias went far beyond just African Americans and women in America. Many different people have felt unaddressed by the medical system. Because of my background, I have always been sympathetic to patients who have been dismissed by the health-care system, but our research has shown Kathy and me that this is not true for all health-care providers.

We selected the title *Dismissed* for our book because it captures the emotion of so many vulnerable people when facing the health-care system. The term "racial and cultural bias" is in the subtitle to add emphasis and clarity. While racial bias is clear to us all, many of us do not really understand the deep effect that ongoing microaggressions can cause. We are appalled by overt racism but fail to see how the steady drip of explicit and implicit bias wears away at the physical, mental, and emotional health of people of color. "Cultural bias" is a broader term that relates to when we use the standards of our own culture to interpret situations, actions, and data from another culture. We make assumptions based on how we are raised, and this leads to bias. For example, there may be cultural differences in how people speak, their religious beliefs, or how they understand ethical concepts or evidence-based proof. We experience cultural bias in every facet of our lives. In public, we may interpret certain gestures or ways of speaking as offensive or rude because they are not used in our own culture. In schools, standardized testing may not consider critical cultural factors. At work, people are treated differently because of cultural standards we have of not only race but weight, age, gender, sexual orientation, and other factors.

By the way, in this book I use the term "doctors," but I am really referring to all members of the health-care team: physician assistants, nurse practitioners, nurses, lab technicians, aides, front office and billing personnel, and so many more. When patients are sick and vulnerable, they have encounters with all these medical team members.

None of my views about bias toward patients changed based on the interviews and research we did for this book. But COVID, and how we have reacted to the pandemic, did affect my perspectives deeply. I watched with pride as the health-care industry rose to the crisis. Doctors and their teams functioned under dangerous, exhausting, and heartwrenching conditions. Public health experts persistently tried to educate people about social distancing and mask-wearing. Scientists and pharmaceutical companies worked tirelessly to find a vaccine and better treatments. But then many people's attitudes toward medical science became politicized. A voter's political affiliation became more important to them than facts. Anti-maskers derided those wearing masks as un-American, despite research clearly showing protective benefits. We were a nation divided and growing very tired of a pandemic that was changing everything. We put our hope in a vaccine, and our prayers were answered. But then came the anti-vaxxers. They were convinced that the science wasn't proven. They insisted that the side effects were horrible. They accepted the gossip "science" that boosting your immune system would work better than vaccines. False information about the vaccines spread. The last straw for me came when I saw seriously sick COVID patients prescribing their own treatment based on what they had read on the internet or heard from friends. Patients were fighting their doctors, while the same doctors were fighting for their patients' lives. This was not the shared decision-making we aim for in our practices. Instead, I saw patients filled with hostility and disrespect for health-care providers.

That's when it hit me. I needed to include the bias against science in this book. It had become a major bias, impacting outcomes in the same way as racial and gender bias. And I knew that I needed to address *what patients must do* to realize and end their own dismissal of health-care professionals.

I have approached this topic as the primary care physician I am. I have taken a holistic and comprehensive approach, leaving the in-depth discussions to specialists. Remember, I am not a psychologist, researcher, policy maker, or hospital administrator. I am a Black woman primary care doctor who grew up in poverty without health insurance. My views are seen through those lenses, and I bring my own biases to the table.

THIS BOOK IS written for both health-care practitioners and patients. It's a bit risky when you approach two distinct audiences who have different knowledge and perspectives, but I feel strongly that one way to bridge the divide is to look at the big picture in a more holistic manner. To that end, some of what I have covered may not be new to you. I hope, however, knitting it together under one framework will provide "aha" moments that encourage dialogue and action.

The book is divided into four sections. The first provides perspectives on vulnerability, compassion, and how doctors approach diagnosis and treatment. We have also included some solutions right up front so you can see that many challenges are solvable. In part 2, we look at specific biases based on race and ethnicity, gender identity and sexual orientation, age, disabilities, and obesity. Part 3 examines several complex challenges, including bias against science, how we pay for services, representation in pharma and research, and technology. We conclude with a section on what we can do right now and ideas for the future.

In addition to including personal and professional stories and other people's research, Kathy and I conducted a public survey. It is not a survey to be considered scientific evidence. Rather, it is a public opinion poll to get a "pulse" on how people from multiple races, genders, body types, economic backgrounds, and ages felt about their interactions with health-care providers. We call it our "Pulse Survey."

To date, more than three hundred people have answered the survey, which included questions such as:

- Have you ever changed doctors because you did not like the way a medical professional treated you?

- What factors made you feel like you were being treated differently by a medical professional?
- If you had a choice of equally competent doctors, would same gender or same race be more important in selecting your physician?
- Who do you feel is most likely to practice empathy when you are undergoing medical treatment?
- What percentage of the time do you feel your current doctor listens to you?
- What percentage of the time do you follow your doctor's treatment instructions?
- What percentage of the time do you feel vulnerable when you are at a medical appointment/procedure?

Our Pulse Survey is ongoing, and so far, more than 75 percent of survey respondents have said they felt that they were not listened to by a current or past medical professional. Even I was surprised by that number. We have included many of our respondents' verbatim comments throughout this book.

If you would like to take this survey, go to https://www.angela marshallmd.com.

Dismissed offers you a picture of the bias problem and its tremendous impact on individuals and society. I hope it also gives you a vision of what we can do to instigate change. To quote the great James Baldwin, African American writer and social critic, "Not everything that is faced can be changed; but nothing can be changed until it is faced."

PART 1

Vulnerable Patients and Doctors

I've learned that people will forget what you said, people will forget what you did, but people will never forget how you made them feel.

—MAYA ANGELOU

CHAPTER 1

How Dismissal Can Lead to Death

T HE DELIVERY OF MY SON Nathan was followed by one of the most harrowing experiences of my life. Once home, I woke up with the worst headache. I mean, the WORST. It was so incredibly severe that I felt like with each pulsation of my heart, someone was beating my head in with a baseball bat. The throbbing was crushing and unbearable, and my face was so swollen that I didn't recognize who I was in the mirror. I looked like some distorted, monstrous version of myself.

My husband immediately took me to the hospital, where I remember the staff asking me repeatedly about the level of my pain. I was totally out of it, but they listened intently to what I was saying and were extremely respectful, helpful, and attentive. I felt cared for and believed they were acting on my behalf without my having to say a word or advocate for myself. I later found out that it required several doses of morphine to make the headache bearable. I was diagnosed with postpartum preeclampsia, which is extremely rare. It had progressed to a very dangerous level and almost caused a stroke. Quite simply, the health-care team in the emergency room cared for me well and saved my life.

Ironically, at the same time I was having my postpartum episode, my precious newborn son was fighting for his life in the NICU. He was born with posterior urethral valves, the same disorder that my first son had, After my firstborn was diagnosed, I researched the disorder and was told that it was very rare and, most important, not genetic. Since the odds that it would happen again were almost nonexistent, my husband and I decided to try for a second child.

During my five-month pregnancy ultrasound, we received shocking news. Not only did our unborn child have the same disorder, but also it was a much more severe case than what my first son had. The condition caused my newborn's kidneys and lungs to develop poorly, resulting in the need for immediate heart and lung support after birth, and dialysis a few days later. After two months in the hospital, Nathan was stable enough to be discharged to home. The goal was to allow him to grow large enough to qualify for a kidney transplant when he was six months old. A world-renowned pediatric kidney specialist at our local children's hospital would follow his progress.

I had just finished my fourth year of medical school with only a one-month rotation left to graduate. Nathan's birth was planned so that I would have nine months off to care for my baby. It was a labor of love to help rehabilitate him back to good health, and he was progressing nicely. He was receiving home dialysis, and physical and occupational therapy. Then one day, when I was getting Nathan ready for his scheduled appointment with the specialist, I noticed he didn't seem like himself. He was unresponsive, staring into space with his eyes crossing in different directions.

I rushed him to the hospital, thankful that he already had an appointment that morning, and called ahead to inform them that something seemed really wrong. After examining him, his doctor stated that Nathan would need to be admitted to the hospital. But the hospital was full, and we would have to wait for a bed and for treatment to start. Although the doctor had Nathan admitted, he didn't seem to feel the urgency that I did. He hadn't seen the eye-crossing thing I had witnessed, although I explained it in great detail. In fact, the doctor looked doubtful.

When Nathan's vitals were checked, I realized he was even sicker than I thought. His respiratory rate was one hundred times per minute, while a normal respiratory rate is between thirty and sixty. I had learned from my pediatrics rotation that the breathing rate in children is an important indicator of illness and one of the most important vital signs of infants. After waiting over half an hour, I began to ask about the status of the room. When were they going to actually start treating my son? I was told they were still waiting for the room. I explained I didn't think we had much time to wait. "How long can he keep breathing at one hundred times per minute?" I asked. Finally, I raised my voice, "He needs help *now!*"

One nurse seemed to understand my urgency. She even expressed her own concerns. She called the doctor, but he kept dismissing both of us. He finally came back into the room and, without examining Nathan, said, "Look, I've been doing this for thirty years. His electrolytes are out of balance because he is sick. But as soon as we get him to a room and give him fluids, we'll get him tanked up, and he'll be back to his normal self in no time."

Something about the doctor reminding me of his thirty years of experience made me breathe a sigh of relief. In fact, I even felt a bit embarrassed that I had been raising my voice. I wanted to advocate for my son, but I did not want to appear ungrateful, nor did I want to overreact. After all, I was a medical student, and he was a doctor who had cared for many very sick children. The doctor had it under control. He was a world-renowned kidney specialist. I even told my husband he could go home and gather our things because it was just a waiting game.

Then the nurse returned to check Nathan one more time. During the exam, my baby stopped breathing. She called a code blue. Nathan's heart had stopped. She told me we had to do CPR. I immediately started breathing into his mouth, crying hysterically. It seemed a lifetime between our starting CPR and the arrival of the code team. I was ushered out of the room and into the hallway, where I prayed harder than I ever have in my life.

Nathan did not make it. My life was shattered. In fact, this is the first time I have publicly written in detail about the events of the worst day of my life. My son's death crushed me. It took a long time to regain my self-esteem, my confidence, my everything. I cannot even find the words to describe how difficult it was to go back to the same hospital to complete my rotation one month after he died, but I had no choice. I knew that no matter how painful, I needed to graduate medical school. I had a mission: to practice medicine in a different way so no one would ever go through what I had.

I don't know why Nathan's doctor dismissed me. I don't know why he would not listen to my repeated concerns. I don't know why he did not see this emergency for what it was: a life-or-death situation. Was it because I was a woman? Was it the color of my skin? Did he not want to be challenged by a med student? Was he burned-out? Was he arrogant because of his past accomplishments? Was he simply having a bad day? I don't know the answer. But every day I feel the loss that resulted from his dismissal of the person who knew Nathan best, his mother.

And I know the guilt. For a very long time, I was mad at myself for backing down when my gut told me what was right. I allowed that doctor to make me feel like an irrational, overly emotional woman— the way many women are made to feel when trying to convey their anxieties or story to someone who will not or cannot accept or understand. It was the most painful lesson I ever learned and the single experience that made me vow to NEVER be that kind of doctor and to ALWAYS listen to my patients.

You may be surprised that after this tragedy and trauma I still wanted to be a doctor. In fact, based on my book title and what I have written so far, you may be wondering why I would even consider medicine as my calling. Here's the truth: I want to heal people. Like me, the vast majority of people go into medicine because they really do want to heal. Most health-care providers are wholeheartedly dedicated to saving lives. You have only to look at our frontline health-care workers during COVID-19 to see the extraordinary heroism of doctors, nurses, lab technicians, physician assistants, nurse practitioners, and the numerous people that support them to know the depth of their commitment.

During times of doubt, I also go back to my personal story of having my life saved by professionals who listened. I probably would not be alive today if my pain had been dismissed and I was not treated for postpartum preeclampsia. The emergency room doctors and nurses listened closely to an extremely vulnerable new mother and responded with respect for me, which led to the right diagnosis and treatment.

The Bias Factor

You cannot really listen to, respect, show empathy for, and believe people if you are operating with an attitude of bias, mistrust, dismissal, or fear. That attitude clouds communication, distorts diagnosis, misdirects treatment, and lessens patient compliance.

Though bias is a central theme of this book, I want to state that I do not believe that the medical community is just a bastion of racists and misogynists. Yes, there are practitioners who believe they are superior to people of color and women, and they show it in their interactions. Yes, there are practitioners who hate and are threatened by men and women who are not heterosexual. Yes, there are practitioners who find obese people disgusting and undisciplined. Yes, there are practitioners who are irritated by elderly patients. But I believe the numbers are not different in health care than in other professions. What is different in health care, however, is that, like in law enforcement, their decisions and actions may make the difference between life and death.

The fact is that patients and health-care providers are human, and ALL humans have biases. These can affect how we listen, observe, and act, and can lead any of us to mistrust and dismiss others.

So, what exactly is bias? Most researchers define bias as our beliefs, thoughts, and feelings that we are either unaware of or that we misunderstand in ourselves. We unconsciously may prefer or have an aversion to a person or group of people, which results in our attitude or stereotype. For example, multiple studies show that without even realizing that they are doing it, people frequently associate Black people with criminality, obese people with laziness, and women with emotionality. These are all biases that can have severe repercussions in health care. That's why we must be vigilant in understanding our biases and reframing our thinking.

Everyone is wired for bias. It is part of what helps us learn quickly and exist in the world. Bias is not a bad word. Yet, unchecked, bias built through learned behaviors and experiences can be highly destructive, since it leads to dismissal and mistrust. For a patient to be treated differently by a medical professional because of their unchecked bias is simply not okay.

People feel bias for multiple reasons. In the Pulse Survey we administered, more than 50 percent of respondents felt they were treated differently by a medical professional because they were female, 35 percent because of their body size, 34 percent because of age, 33 percent because of race, 22 percent because of ethnicity, and 5 percent because they identified as LGBTQIA.

The World of "Isms"

We live in a world where "isms" and "phobias" are a common part of our language. Some people will scoff and say everyone is just being "too sensitive." I do not agree. Dismissal of people because of who they are is just plain wrong and, in health care, can be deadly. Awareness and education are critical as we try to curb the effect of bias.

It's also important to remember that many people are faced with multiple isms. An older person can be dealing with ageism, ableism, and mentalism. If you then add racism and sexism, then you have an intense list of stressors that affect health. To add some clarity, let's start with a common, but not exhaustive, list of bias-driven terms and definitions:

Racism: Discrimination against people of color because of their race.

Sexism: Discrimination against women and girls because of their sex.

Ableism: Discrimination against people with disabilities.

Ageism: Discrimination against older populations because of their age.

Mentalism: Discrimination against people with a mental trait or condition.

Elitism: Discrimination against people because of their "lack of" education, money, or job status.

Denialism: Denying the validity of something despite proof or strong evidence that it is valid.

Homophobia: Discrimination against nonheterosexual people because of their sexuality.

Transphobia: Discrimination against trans people or gender nonconforming people because of their gender identity.

Xenophobia: Discrimination against people from other countries.

Fatphobia: Discrimination against people because of their size.

Bias against Women

I am particularly sensitive to bias against women since I have spent my whole career focusing on women's health. As an internal medicine doctor, I have a keen interest in women and realize that many women prefer women doctors. Very early in my career, I felt that women needed special attention to their health. That's why I started my practice, Comprehensive Women's Health.

I cannot tell you how many times I have heard women patients tell me about male doctors who said, "It sounds like anxiety" when there was really something going on physically. We all know the stereotype: Men don't listen to women. From the boardroom to the bedroom, they often fail to hear or take what women say seriously.

Men also see health differently than women. We make half-hearted jokes about it all the time. For example, the concept of the "man cold." When women have a cold, they are considered whiny when they complain of feeling badly. They are expected to work and take care of the home and kids. Empathy is not on the table. However, when men have a cold, somehow the world stops to give them care, support, and sympathy. Oh boy, you may have just seen my own bias showing up!

But on a serious note, what really happens when women are not listened to about health matters? It can be detrimental and sometimes deadly. Why? First, we present with different symptoms from various diseases than men. How we "present" means what a doctor is looking for physically and verbally when you go to them for a problem.

Too often women are dismissed and ultimately have worse outcomes than men because the medical community is looking for "male symptoms," whereas we have "female symptoms." Many of our symptoms are less precise physically and vaguer. For example, heart disease in women can present with chest pain as it does in men, but the next most common complaints from women having a heart attack are fatigue, anxiety, and shortness of breath. With these symptoms many women are dismissed and told to simply get rest, or that their heart troubles are likely just anxiety. Take a Xanax and go home. This is why the mortality rate for women with heart disease is worse than for men.

Since women's symptoms are so different than what medical training teaches us, I learned firsthand that the most important skill for a doctor treating a woman is *to listen*. The second thing I have learned is *to believe them*. If a patient complains of a side effect from a medication that is not listed on the package insert, I pay attention. I take her off the medication to see if the side effect goes away. If I want to know beyond the shadow of a doubt, I reintroduce the medicine to see if side effects reoccur. If they do, I have my answer.

Let's spend a few moments seeing how listening and believing relate to heart disease and women. I want to use heart disease to illustrate how bias specifically is destroying the health of our mothers and daughters, wives and lovers, nieces and best friends.

Heart disease is the leading cause of death in women and men. Women, however, are more likely to die. A study published in the *New England Journal of Medicine* found that women are seven times more likely than men to be misdiagnosed and discharged in the middle of having a heart attack. Why? Because the medical expectations of how most diseases look are based on male physiology, but women have altogether different symptoms when having a heart attack. These differences extend to heart disease in general, as you can see from the following two examples from my own practice.

Ms. Williams came to me complaining about shortness of breath. She was about to get on a plane the next day for her brother's funeral in Arizona. She had told her male cardiologist about the problem, but he had discounted her concerns because she'd had a normal stress test six months earlier. When I saw her, she was visibly short of breath, even though her oxygen level was normal. I remember the day well because it was one of the busiest of my career, a day when I saw twenty-nine patients nonstop. I called her cardiologist and insisted that she get a heart catheterization. He was able to get her scheduled for the very next morning. Unfortunately, I had to advise her that she had to miss the funeral. That was a tough decision for both of us.

Upon examination, she was found to have four blood vessels that were almost 100 percent blocked. It was so severe that they took her straight to open-heart surgery. I often wondered what would have happened had she not brought this up to me? Or if I had put off that phone call to the cardiologist because of my patient load? Had her cardiologist taken the time to really listen to her? Did he know she was a woman who rarely complained? Did he dismiss her symptom of shortness of breath because she didn't have any chest pain?

Another patient had a similar experience when her male cardiologist told her that she was fine, even though she, too, was having progressive shortness of breath. I sent her to a lung specialist, who said her lungs were fine. Then I sent Andrea to another cardiologist who looked at her risk factors, including diabetes, obesity, and high stress, and told her she needed to exercise more and lose weight. He also suggested she engage in meditation to relieve stress.

By this time, I was getting frustrated and angry, as was Andrea, so I sent her to a third cardiologist, who happened to be a woman. This time I called and advocated for her, but I didn't need to, because the cardiologist immediately understood what I was concerned about and took my patient seriously. Upon catheterization, it was found that she had one vessel that was over 95 percent blocked, requiring an immediate stent to open it up to restore the blood flow. We had finally found a specialist who did not bring her own bias to the table and actually listened.

I cannot tell you how critical it is that women understand heart attack symptoms and how to advocate for themselves. It can save their lives or those of others. Kathy, my co-author, was sitting at a birthday dinner in a restaurant with a close family member. The birthday girl, a woman in her early seventies with no history of heart disease in her family, started feeling nauseous and light-headed. She complained of being short of breath but attributed it to her asthma. At no point did she feel any pain or pressure in her chest or arms, which are the classic signs of a heart attack in men.

She wanted to stay at the birthday dinner because she was sure that "it would pass." Her dinner companions, however, insisted that they leave. When they got back to her home, the ill woman planned to go to bed and have her family members leave her alone. Because Kathy and I had talked about symptom, she was suspicious that her relative might be experiencing a heart attack. Against her relative's wishes, she called 911, who immediately dispatched an ambulance. Even though it arrived in just a few moments, by the time she was on her way to the hospital, she was experiencing chest pains. She *was* having a heart attack. If her dinner companions had allowed her to dismiss her symptoms, it is questionable if they would have celebrated her birthday the following year. Their knowledge and persistence saved her life.

ANOTHER AREA OF medical bias for women is around pain. Medical professionals often underestimate the levels of pain a woman is experiencing or even insist she is making her symptoms up. Too often they categorize these women as being hypochondriacs. Interestingly, hypochondria in ancient Greece and during the medieval period was perceived as a male disease, while women were diagnosed with hysteria. During the seventeenth and eighteenth centuries, men were thought to experience hypochondria from too much use of their brains, while women's hysteria was because they were "delicate" and had "nerve weakness."

Later, health anxiety in women became associated with their desire for attention. We can thank Sigmund Freud for that theory. What then developed was the routine disbelieving of women's pain and undervaluing or dismissing their complaints. Statistics back this up: Women in pain are much more likely than men to receive prescriptions for sedatives rather than pain medication. Women wait an average of sixty-five minutes before receiving an analgesic for acute abdominal pain in the ER in the United States, while men wait only forty-nine minutes. Seventy percent of people impacted by chronic pain are women, yet 80 percent of pain studies are conducted on male mice or human men.

Bias Based on Race

Recently I was asked if, as an African American and a woman, I would choose to go to an African American male or a White woman doctor. As a doctor and outspoken advocate for other women, I was surprised how quickly and definitively I responded. I would select a male African American versus a White woman doctor if both were equally competent. Where did my bias come from? It is driven by both statistics and emotions.

Quite simply, I have lots of statistics that show me that a White-dominated health system has failed my brothers and sisters quite spectacularly. Racial and ethnic biases have had dramatic consequences that have led to a disparity in the health care delivered to Americans. According to the *2018 National Health Care Quality and Disparities Report*, disparities persist, especially for uninsured populations living in poverty. African Americans, Native Americans, Alaska Natives (AI/ANs), and Native Hawaiians/Pacific Islanders (NHPIs) received worse care than Whites for about 40 percent of quality measures. Hispanics received worse care than Whites for about 35 percent of quality measures. Simply put, African Americans and other minority groups in the U.S. experience more illness, worse outcomes, and premature death compared with Whites. Black Americans die at a younger age than White Americans from diseases such as heart disease, stroke, cancer, asthma, and diabetes.

The Black infant mortality rate is more than two times higher than for Whites: 11.4 deaths per 1,000 live births for Blacks compared with 4.9 for Whites. Black women are more than three times as likely as

White women to die of childbirth-related causes, according to the Centers for Disease Control and Prevention (40.8 per 100,000 births compared to 12.7).

On an emotional level, I believe, like many African Americans, that no matter what my professional, economic, and social status, I will be subjected to stereotyping by race. I believe that because so many White people are unaware of both their implicit and explicit biases that I will be talked to differently, listened to differently, diagnosed differently, and treated differently by a White doctor versus a Black doctor.

Every day as an African American I experience racism. It is so part of my life that it is the lens through which I see interactions professionally and personally. As a mother of a son, I know that he is way more at risk than his White counterparts for violence and imprisonment from American institutions. I have experienced fear in my life for my family and myself because of the color of my skin. So if I can find a doctor who shares my heritage, why wouldn't I make that choice? Rationally, I know that most physicians are not racist and are committed to treating all patients equally. However, I also know they operate in an inherently racist, White-dominated system.

Emotionally, I also cannot and will never forget American history and how medicine used people of color badly. And we are not talking centuries ago. In Puerto Rico, women were sterilized in the name of population control from the 1930s to the 1970s. As a result of the Family Planning Services and Population Research Act of 1970, close to 25 percent of Native American women were also sterilized. The government-sanctioned Tuskegee experiments from 1932 to 1972 infected African American men with syphilis without informed consent or adequate treatment, despite the study's leading to the discovery that penicillin was effective.

Now let's go back to the issue of pain. The medical community systematically dismissed pain in women, but it bought into myths about African Americans and pain at even more frightening levels. As recently as 2016, in a study published in the *Proceedings of the National Academies of Science*, 40 percent of first- and second-year medical students endorsed the belief that "Black people's skin is thicker than White people's." Furthermore, those students who believed that Black people are not as sensitive to pain as White people were less likely to treat Black people's pain appropriately. Additionally, a meta-analysis of twenty years of studies covering many sources of pain in numerous settings found African American patients were 22 percent less likely than White patients to receive any pain medication.

So based on statistics and emotions, I would feel more comfortable being treated by an African American doctor. I acknowledge that bias in myself. Unfortunately, the likelihood of finding that doctor is not very high, since just 5 percent of doctors in America are African American. While increasing the number of African American doctors is an important goal, we cannot count on that as the only solution. Instead, recognizing and erasing the prejudices that permeate health care must be the priority. To fight racism and discrimination, we need to be open to identifying and controlling biases. We need to be able to overcome overt bigotry, learn from it, and educate others. Each of us must do our part as individuals, but we also need to make changes in institutional policy and medical education.

Let me also be very clear. Racism is not an issue exclusively for African Americans. This is simply the area I feel most qualified to talk about because of my own background and research. But rest assured, racism exists for many ethnic groups of Americans. I will share some perspectives on health care in regard to the Native American, Latinx, and Asian American populations also.

Racial and cultural bias exists not just in doctors toward patients. I know of Black doctors who are wary of setting up practices outside of large cities because they are concerned that in more homogenously White environments, other doctors will not refer to them and patients will not seek their services. I remember my own experiences in Indiana, where some people didn't believe I was really a practicing physician. They thought, "Black and a woman? No way can she be a real doctor." They could not see me as an educated professional. Contrast that to my later move to Washington, DC, where people looked at my last name and asked if I was related to Supreme Court Judge Thurgood Marshall. In that urban environment, being an accomplished African American was normal.

On a more dramatic level, physicians have been insulted and even threatened because they are Muslim or Jewish. Health-care providers have been attacked because of the color of their skin. Racist patients exist and are becoming more vocal. They need to be dealt with in the same way we need to address racism in the workplace and our communities—with strong actions and strong voices.

Other Types of Biases

There are other biases threatening the health of Americans. Perhaps the most difficult one to deal with currently is the bias against science. One of the most visible anti-science movements has focused on discrediting vaccines. This has become a life-and-death issue with diseases like COVID-19. In a country at war over the validity of vaccinations, masks, and social distancing, how can people identify or change their biases against science, a discipline that has saved the lives of millions?

We need to end our bias against our own ability for self-care and embrace our responsibility to listen to and believe in our bodies. I cannot tell you how many times I have seen a patient who said, "It's been bothering me for months, but I didn't think it was a big deal." Your body knows and tells you things. You just need to pay attention. This does not mean that you need to go into the hypervigilant mode of a hypochondriac, a person who is convinced that they have a serious illness no matter how minor the symptom. But I will tell you this: In my career I have met many more patients who underestimated their symptoms than those who overestimated. So just listen and believe what your body is telling you with its extreme fatigue or thirst, unusual pain, or changes in your skin, vision, and bodily functions. That's a big part of learning how to heal yourself, as well as how to communicate when getting help from medical professionals.

I also want to share with you thoughts on what is known as "blame bias." Blame bias is when we blame the person, not their environment or circumstances. There has been a lot of discussion of this idea in management and leadership coaching, but I believe it has a great deal of relevance to health care. Our society sometimes attributes the good and bad of a person's health solely to their lifestyle issues. "He got lung cancer. I thought that was impossible since he wasn't a smoker." Or "I'm sure all her health problems would go away if she only lost weight." This attribution of blame can be found both in health-care providers and patients. For patients, it leads to guilt and a feeling of "Is this all my fault?" Blame bias leans health-care providers toward making false judgments based on biased assumptions about patients, who then feel they can't trust the provider.

The Importance of an Oath

Earlier in this chapter, I told you that my passion to heal people has never left me, even though I am seriously dissatisfied with our health-care system and society for their prejudices, biases, and outright racism, which are destroying the health of so many vulnerable people. Along with many other health-care professionals, I have been disheartened by the pandemic. So many of us are simply exhausted, absolutely bewildered and angry at people's failure to take the simple precautions needed to stay out of the hospital.

No matter what, one thing I always remember is that I have taken an oath, the Hippocratic oath. For those of you who do not know about the Hippocratic oath, it is a voluntary vow that doctors take to uphold certain ethical standards. Originating in ancient Greece, the modern version of the Hippocratic oath was written in 1964 by Louis Lasagna, dean of the School of Medicine at Tufts University. It goes like this:

I swear to fulfill, to the best of my ability and judgment, this covenant:

I will respect the hard-won scientific gains of those physicians in whose steps I walk, and gladly share such knowledge as is mine with those who are to follow.

I will apply, for the benefit of the sick, all measures [that] are required, avoiding those twin traps of overtreatment and therapeutic nihilism.

I will remember that there is art to medicine as well as science, and that warmth, sympathy, and understanding may outweigh the surgeon's knife or the chemist's drug.

I will not be ashamed to say, "I know not," nor will I fail to call in my colleagues when the skills of another are needed for a patient's recovery.

I will respect the privacy of my patients, for their problems are not disclosed to me that the world may know. Most especially must I tread with care in matters of life and death. If it is given me to save a life, all thanks. But it may also be within my power to take a life; this awesome responsibility must be faced with great humbleness and awareness of my own frailty. Above all, I must not play at God.

I will remember that I do not treat a fever chart, a cancerous growth, but a sick human being, whose illness may affect the person's family and economic stability. My responsibility includes these related problems, if I am to care adequately for the sick.

I will prevent disease whenever I can, for prevention is preferable to cure.

I will remember that I remain a member of society, with special obligations to all my fellow human beings, those sound of mind and body as well as the infirm.

If I do not violate this oath, may I enjoy life and art, respected while I live and remembered with affection thereafter. May I always act so as to preserve the finest traditions of my calling, and may I long experience the joy of healing those who seek my help.

As you can see, there is no direct mention of bias in the Hippocratic oath. Yet for me, its words clearly indicate that we need to not harm those whom we have sworn to help heal. "I will remember that I remain a member of society, with special obligations to all my fellow human beings, those sound of mind and body as well as the infirm." *All my fellow human beings*—inclusive words that show us all as equally human. In medical school, I remember seeing people in the hospital who had just committed crimes and were handcuffed to a bed with a security guard outside. It wasn't always easy, but we treated each and every one of these patients as human beings, not criminals. They received great care, and the doctors never acted as if they weren't "worthy." In fact, we were probably as attentive to them as their defense attorneys. My maternal grandmother was one of those health-care providers who worked in a prison. She often shared stories about her patients and how she strived to care for them in a nonjudgmental manner. She once told me that she never asked them what crime got them imprisoned and that the inmates had affectionately started calling her "Mother Love."

Biases flourish when we forget that we are all more alike than different. Biases flourish when we think in an "either/or" mindset instead of a "both/and" mindset. Biases flourish when we forget the power of education, dialogue, and positive action to unite us against the real threats: disease and death. Biases close our minds and allow us to dismiss others. They cause physical, emotional, and spiritual destruction. In contrast, empathy and listening let us encourage living. Let us choose life together. And the first place to start is to acknowledge our own vulnerability to bias, both as patients and health-care providers.

CHAPTER 2

We're All Vulnerable

VULNERABILITY IN A DOCTOR'S OFFICE is not rare. In fact, 50 per-cent of the people who answered our survey said that they felt vulnerable when they were at a medical appointment or procedure.

Pain. Fear. Mistrust. Those three emotions serve as the foundation of vulnerability in patients. When you are sick, or even just trying to live in this chaotic world of the pandemic, you are at your most vul-nerable. Unfortunately, despite your state of vulnerability, decisions still need to be made about tests and treatment or preventative ac-tions like vaccines and medication. These decisions require either your own consent or that of your family, if you are incapacitated. It's hard to make those decisions when you're full of pain, fear, and mis-trust. At these vulnerable moments, you are asked to trust that your doctor and other health-care providers will provide you with the best treatment based on data. You are asked to trust that they are follow-ing established medical protocols that will give you the best outcome.

I don't think there is anyone more vulnerable than a patient in pain. Sometimes it is physical pain. Other times it is emotional pain, like the kind that made me vulnerable when my son was ill. In those moments of pain, the ways health-care professionals and patients see and relate to each other often set the course of health outcomes. Their views of each other and their communication (or the lack of it) can determine the choices they make in giving and receiving medical care.

It is not hard to imagine this vulnerability because you have probably experienced it yourself. You are in a doctor's office telling intimate details that you never discuss with anyone. Perhaps you are even naked for an exam. You are worried and scared about what is wrong with you. Your body hurts, and your mind is racing. You don't want to be there, but you are. We are talking serious vulnerability. Most people can relate to this feeling.

Vulnerability and Pain

Marianne is a patient of mine with a history of childhood polio who has been in a wheelchair since childhood. She epitomizes a vulnerable patient. She suffers from chronic pain in her limbs, which are severely atrophied due to her condition. I referred her to a pain management clinic, which treated her with opioids in a controlled setting. I made that referral because it is almost impossible for a primary physician like me to manage pain with powerful drugs, since it requires constant monitoring and specific expertise.

As part of the standard protocol, during each visit the pain clinic tests patients for recreational drugs, as well as those prescribed, to make sure the person is taking the medication and not using other drugs. In Marianne's case, she was taking her medicine correctly but had run out a few days before her visit because the clinic had reduced the quantity of pills they gave her. Since she used a wheelchair, they did not check her urine for drug levels, but instead did a cheek swab.

Her result revealed no illicit drugs but showed no presence of the prescribed drug in her system, either. Based on the cheek-swab test, the office manager assumed that Marianne had not been taking her medication. He told her that she could no longer be a patient and was being dropped from the clinic. When she asked why, she was told that because she didn't have the medication in her system, the pain clinic believed she was selling her medication. When she explained that she had run out of pills, they did not believe her. They also wrote a very negative account in her medical records, which would now follow her into any other medical practice.

I called the clinic and told them their assessment was absolutely wrong. I then referred Marianne to a new pain doctor and personally called to explain the situation and vouch for her, saying she is over sixty-five years old and uses a wheelchair. I said I had known her for many years, and she had never shown any signs of drug abuse or selling pain medication.

Why did the first pain clinic assume that this highly vulnerable patient was selling drugs? I believe it was a combination of biases: she was an African American woman, overweight, older, and in a wheelchair with chronic pain. Would they have come to the same conclusion if she had been a White, affluent professional male? I just don't think so. This is one of the most serious mistreatments of a very vulnerable patient that I have ever seen.

It is also important to note that once Marianne was discharged from one pain management clinic, particularly with what they had put in her record, she would likely have been blacklisted from other pain clinics. Marianne would have lived a life of horrible chronic pain. She may have had to turn to street drugs, which are very dangerous and expensive.

I absolutely understand that because the laws are so tough, doctors don't want to take the risk of prescribing pain medicine for anyone who they perceive might be abusing or selling. But compassion, respect, and common sense are needed. Those doctors' perceptions of their patients may be unfounded, or built on bias. The first pain clinic failed to look at Marianne as a human being and made false and accusatory assumptions, possibly based on her race and physical conditions.

Fortunately, I was able to find another doctor to manage her pain, and Marianne is still under their care. But what happens to vulnerable patients in pain who do not have a doctor advocate? One of the things I most often see in those patients is disengagement.

Vulnerability and Disengagement

When vulnerable people encounter health-care professionals who mistreat them, they may disengage, stop going to the doctor altogether, and resort to their own devices. Often, they become their own Doctor Google and become natural herb and supplement administrators. This DIY approach to health care hurts patients. They try to analyze data and make medical recommendations for themselves. The problem is that most people do not have the skills to analyze scientific data effectively and often make medical decisions based on misinformation from non-credible sources.

I see too many of these patients at Comprehensive Women's Health. They are women who disconnected from previous health care and have not seen their former doctors for years. They became so disillusioned by an incident with a health-care provider that they stay away from having regular physicals or getting necessary tests like mammograms. Too often, they are not practicing self-care in general, like getting enough sleep, exercising, and watching what they eat. Essentially, they are playing Russian roulette with their health. As a result, I see them when they haven't avoided the bullet. They have a disease or condition that could have been prevented or managed with less intervention than they now need.

Then there are the patients who have excellent relationships with their doctors but disengage because they have stopped trusting the person who is the medical expert. This one always frustrates me. We don't practice this kind of behavior with other professionals. Imagine standing over the plumber in your house and telling them what size pipe to use. Or explaining to your tax accountant exactly which deductions would be most advantageous to you. Or interrupting your lawyer during a trial and complaining that she is using a wrong argument.

But when it comes to health, so important to their quality of life, many people ignore the advice of their doctors. Let me give you some examples from my own patients, most of whom have been with me for many years and rate me highly.

Hannah consistently resisted getting a flu shot, but finally got one in October. The following February, she got sick with a viral illness that was probably a severe cold. The next year when it was time for another flu shot, she blamed her illness on the vaccine, saying, "Last time I got that flu shot I got really sick!" Perhaps Hannah had heard from the grapevine that vaccines make you sick. I had to remind her that her sickness was several months after the vaccination and certainly not caused by it. It took a lot of time and energy, two very limited resources for a primary doctor, to convince her.

Ms. Williams had severe hypertension but resisted taking medication. Over time, her blood pressure got so incredibly high that she finally agreed to drug treatment. Soon after, additional tests showed that her kidneys were damaged. Did she blame her kidney failure on the years of untreated hypertension? No, she blamed it on the medication, which would have prevented the kidney damage if she had taken it when she really needed to.

And still another patient recently told me that she would not get the COVID vaccine because she didn't trust it. Jesse shared that a friend of hers got the vaccine and was admitted to the hospital for diabetes complications. Instead of realizing that her friend's hospital admission was because of her out-of-control diabetes, my patient blamed it on the COVID vaccine. I could not convince her otherwise, no matter what data I shared with her.

In the last century, most Americans had strong confidence in our medical system. Those numbers have gone down, according to most pollsters. Fortunately, individual doctors fare better. In a January 2019 Pew Research Center survey, 74 percent of Americans said they had a mostly positive view of doctors. Around half of Americans said medical doctors always or usually care about their patients' best interests (57 percent), do a good job providing diagnoses and treatment recommendations (49 percent), and provide fair and accurate information when making recommendations (48 percent).

Actually, I don't like those numbers all that much. Less than half of those surveyed believe we are doing a good job providing diagnoses and treatment recommendations? I guess that's a better number than a major league baseball pitcher, but I can tell you that for most doctors that is a morale killer. Our ability to help people is the number one motivator for us. Most doctors would not be satisfied with only half of their patients thinking they were doing a good job.

Health Equality vs. Health Equity

Often when we find population disparities in health care, it is because of inequities in those populations' social and health histories. Those inequities make those populations more vulnerable in health-care situations. But what is *inequity*, versus the *equality* that we all grew up knowing we needed to aim for?

Many of us grew up learning that *equality* is the goal of social change, particularly for people of color and women. In the schoolroom, we learned about the Civil Rights Movement, which demanded *equality* for African Americans, and the *Equal* Rights Amendment (ERA), a proposed amendment to the U.S. Constitution that would invalidate many state and federal laws that discriminate against women. We have often used the words *equality* and *equity* interchangeably, since there are many similarities between the two.

But the people who work in the social justice world have helped us understand the difference. Let me share definitions from the

Annie E. Casey Foundation, a private philanthropy, based in Baltimore, that provides grants to help improve educational, economic, social and health outcomes for children and young people:

> Equity involves trying to understand and give people what they need to enjoy full, healthy lives. Equality, in contrast, aims to ensure that everyone gets the same things in order to enjoy full, healthy lives. Like equity, equality aims to promote fairness and justice, but it can only work if everyone starts from the same place and needs the same things.

When I am talking about a patient's vulnerability in a medical setting, that patient may very well be starting at a different place than other patients—*inequity*—because of their specific situation. While two patients might both feel vulnerability, one may be sicker or more fearful, and so more vulnerable, because of who they are, where they live, and how they grew up. As medical professionals, we need to be aware of that patient's background in order to provide treatment that is *equitable* to that particular patient's needs. As we all know, all patient's backgrounds are not created equal. And often we see patterns of vulnerability in particular populations, defined by race, gender, minority, or socioeconomic status.

Vulnerability and Populations

Up to this point, I have talked primarily about vulnerability and the individual. One area that has been studied extensively over the last twenty years is the vulnerabilities of specific populations. Countless research studies have highlighted disparate health outcomes for vulnerable populations. These groups include racial, ethnic, and religious minorities; women; individuals living in poverty; individuals with chronic diseases and disabilities; seniors; individuals who identify as LGBTQIA; patients who are obese; and others. There's a high likelihood that you fit in at least one of these population groups.

We hear a lot these days about "health disparities" among different populations, especially among minorities. What exactly are health disparities? The Centers for Disease Control and Prevention (CDC) defines health disparities as "preventable differences in the burden of disease, injury, violence, or opportunities to achieve optimal health that are experienced by socially disadvantaged populations."

The Office of Disease Prevention and Health Promotion (ODPHP) explains, "Although the term *disparities* is often interpreted to mean racial or ethnic disparities, many dimensions of disparity exist in the United States, particularly in health. If a health outcome is seen to a greater or lesser extent between populations, there is disparity. Race or ethnicity, sex, sexual identity, age, disability, socioeconomic status, and geographic location all contribute to an individual's ability to achieve good health."

Health disparities do not come from nowhere. They are tied directly to social determinants of health, which include genetics, health behaviors, social and environmental conditions, and access to health care. Social determinants of health shape individuals' health behaviors and are primary drivers of health outcomes.

Health disparities are driven by social and economic inequities that are rooted in racism. This makes vulnerability a huge issue for African Americans. If we are mistreated by medical professionals when in our most vulnerable state as patients, we feel like disengaging from those in power. This is similar to how minority populations feel about the police: When we are mistreated by the police, we feel the need to disengage from them and their authority. The same is true in health care.

Addressing disparities is important not only for social justice but also to improve our health-care system. This book cannot even begin to prescribe the changes needed to address the social determinants of health. That would mean advocating for major changes to address inequities in education, poverty, housing, and a host of other factors. But as patients and health-care providers working on our own behavior and relationships, we can act.

Vulnerability and Disengagement in African Americans

Often when a patient mistrusts doctors, they will dismiss medical recommendations and disengage from those who offer them. Because African Americans have been grievously wronged by medical doctors and scientists throughout history, I think there is a confirmation bias that now exists within our communities that makes us wary of medical recommendations even if they would be of benefit—or might even save lives. And because of history, there's a lot of emotion on this issue, which affects our thinking and reasoning.

As Black people, we have a deep mistrust of many parts of American society, and our health-care system and medical research are at the top of the list. A major contributor to our skepticism is the USPHS Syphilis Study at Tuskegee, a forty-year experiment on African American men that was an atrocity against our people. The Tuskegee experiment finally ended, but medical racism did not. In 2021, research shows that as many of 15 percent of Black women feel mistreated in health-care settings. This perceived mistreatment is palpable among many Black women and has led to many disengaging from the health-care system.

Our disengagement makes us vulnerable. If we seek medical care only when our lives are on the line, we miss out on preventative care and put our health in jeopardy. It creates a collective vulnerability in our community.

Many African Americans have disengaged from the health-care system for all non-life-threatening care and instead opted for a do-it-yourself approach, which in their minds is often more "natural."

Many take vitamins, believing that there is evidence that they can keep illness away. Many take herbal remedies or other therapies that are not scientifically backed.

This do-it-yourself health attitude can include our taking an anecdotal approach in our personal medical "research." "Anecdotal" is defined as being a personal account rather than a fact or research. That means it is not necessarily true or reliable. We might hear stories about treatments from friends, Google, or YouTube and think that if that person had good luck with it, maybe it will work for me. But anecdotal "evidence" comes from just a few individuals' reported success stories. In fact, those few people may have experienced just a placebo effect. The placebo effect means that if you think a regimen will work, it does work because your mind interacts with your body to make it so. This is why medical research often factors in the placebo effect. In medicine, we conduct randomized controlled trials of new treatments on large numbers of people to make sure that new medicines aren't working just because a few people believe in them. We want to make sure that they work better than a placebo. The placebo effect might have made that treatment work for that one guy you saw on Facebook, but that doesn't mean it will work for everybody (or even for anybody else).

In do-it-yourself health, oftentimes patients want facts to support their beliefs but end up veering away from science, toward rumors and scams. This phenomenon played out all too well in the COVID pandemic among many vulnerable populations. For example, at the beginning, many Black folks were saying that we couldn't get COVID. Then there was a prevention and treatment option that went viral, involving boiling water on top of a stove. I had so many people asking me almost daily, "What about this remedy? Does this work?" Yet, when I recommended hand washing and social distancing, perhaps it wasn't robust or exciting enough. The scam remedies were more inviting.

Once the vaccines became available, many of us did not want to have any part of them. Some people claimed that they were allergic, or that immune-system issues prevented them from getting the vaccine. The tables were turned: The patients were telling the doctor why they should not get the shot, instead of the patient asking the doctor, "I have this preexisting condition. Can I still get the vaccine?" The doctor-patient relationship shifted even further apart, resulting in our community's disengagement from health providers and furthering our social vulnerability. Now, even though almost 100 percent of those with deadly COVID symptoms are unvaccinated, a large percentage of the public remains steadfast in their position to not vaccinate.

Because of their vulnerability and mistrust, many patients cannot accept medical recommendations that are good for them. As healthcare providers, we have to do more to build trust. For the African American community, that means graduating more Black doctors, requiring cultural competencies for physicians, tying outcomes and health disparity data to quality and payment incentives, and creating community partnerships with churches and other trusted community advocates.

The Paradox: Doctors Can Be Vulnerable, Too

The paradox is that doctors can be vulnerable too. While most research focuses on patient vulnerability and vulnerability among different patient populations, doctors and other health-care professionals also experience vulnerability. There are many factors involved: work overload, excessive working hours, sleep deprivation, repeated exposure to emotionally charged situations, and dealing with difficult patients.

Yes, I've seen the health-care system evolve over the past years into something that I am not always proud of. And, yes, just like there are good cops and bad cops, there are good health-care providers, and there are those who are not. There are lots of reasons for this, but there are also potential solutions. But first, vulnerability among doctors is a real thing that must be acknowledged.

Let's talk specifically about primary care. There has been a shortage of primary care physicians, exacerbated by the baby boomer generation coming of Medicare age. The primary care shortage was evident even back in the 1990s, but after the baby boomers reached retirement age, the shortage became more pronounced. This shortage has created a strain on the system, resulting in unnecessary patient illness and deaths. A recent study found that having an adequate number of primary care doctors could save an estimated seven thousand lives each year and boost life expectancy by an average of fifty-six days,

We doctors have experienced a considerable burden in trying to keep our patients healthy and alive. A big contributor to our vulnerability is simply the nature of our work. Dr. Sonali Mantoo, a critical care physician, explains that physicians are trained to recognize discomfort in patients, but not their own pain. Additionally, doctors are not trained well to cope with death, medical errors, or malpractice suits. "These very issues are what perpetuate a toxic culture leading to dropout, burnout, and more. We are tested on our Intelligence Quotient. What about our Emotional Quotient?"

At no time has our vulnerability as doctors been more tested than during the pandemic. We lived through a relentless phase, where we did our best to help our patients. Covered from head to toe in personal protective gear, we practiced medicine while literally fearing for our lives. And it was a legitimate fear. At least 115,000 health-care workers worldwide are estimated to have lost their lives to COVID-19, according to the World Health Organization (WHO).

And then came the vaccines, a scientifically validated and tested solution that we saw as the light at the end of the tunnel. Unfortunately, so many Americans saw the vaccines as the devil. In a few moments, I will paint a candid picture for you of what it was like to practice medicine during the pandemic and the months that followed.

For me, there is no better way to talk about doctor vulnerability. And please remember, my amazing staff and I were practicing private primary care. We were not even on the front lines in hospitals, watching countless people die as we feared for our own lives.

We Are All Vulnerable under COVID

The COVID pandemic exposed a lot of vulnerabilities on both sides of the health-care system, doctors and patients. It placed additional pressure on already-stressed-out medical workers. Health inequities existed long before the pandemic, but COVID exacerbated them and led to further disengagement, illness, and death in vulnerable patients.

Primary care is grueling. Generally, we see twenty to thirty patients daily and then have to find time to review test results, communicate them to the patients, handle patient requests that come by phone or email, and deal with insurance forms, pre-authorizations, and other administrative paperwork. For those of us in private practice, we also have to handle insurance denials, collection, and billing headaches. It is not a job for the faint of heart. Even before the pandemic, doctors were overworked and burned-out, with many of my peers strategizing for an early retirement or alternate career. We were hanging by our chin hairs before the pandemic, and COVID was a potential knockout punch, though many still rose to the occasion.

I remember when COVID first began in Wuhan. I watched the news intently, looking for signs to predict where this thing was going. Once I saw it sweep across Europe, especially Italy, I knew for sure that it was only a matter of time before we were hit in the U.S. I posted on social media, warning people to get necessary supplies because it was very likely that we'd have a lockdown of some sort. Many people followed my suggestions; others laughed them off in disbelief. There are people who thank me to this day for my recommendations because they were able to get hand sanitizer or toilet paper in time.

As a doctor, though, I can honestly say we were ill-prepared. Now, I had a doomsday stash for my family (I've always been a strong emergency-preparedness nut), but I was not prepared to handle a global pandemic. There was nothing in medical school to prepare me for this. I had read about the 1918 flu but didn't realize the sheer extent of it, nor the duration of that pandemic and its historical significance. Despite my initial shock, I, along with my team, sprang into action.

The first days were tough. We were constantly tuned in to the CDC for guidance. Thankfully, our practice had acquired a telehealth system three years earlier, a platform that allowed video visit appointments. As a former engineer, I had been super excited about technology like telemedicine in health care, but we had been surprised that our patients didn't share our enthusiasm. We hadn't used the telemedicine platform much, largely due to low patient demand for it. But when the pandemic hit, at least we were already prepared with the technology, if not emotionally ready for the impact of the virus.

We were ready, so we were able to pivot to video appointments. On March 13, 2020, we saw 100 percent of our patients in person. The next business day, Monday, March 16, we saw 50 percent in person and 50 percent by video. And on March 17, we saw 100 percent of our patients via video visit. We did not miss a day of patient care in this transition. On that first day of all-video visits, we evaluated three patients who tested positive for COVID. It was crazy. I was seeing videos of sick patients back-to-back, many of them wrapped in blankets in their beds or shivering and coughing continuously. It was scary.

We also had issues with testing. It wasn't clear what was needed for testing. We were ready to do testing but were getting mixed messages. We were told that labs needed a doctor's order. We had to figure out what test we were ordering. I have to say that LabCorp of America was super helpful. They were right in the trenches, developing the test and providing us with swabs and viral culture tubes early on.

Then it got much worse. Two months after the shutdown of America, George Floyd was murdered. The intersection of COVID and

Black Lives Matter increased not only my own sense of vulnerability but that of my patients, many of whom are African American women.

The racial inequity around COVID magnified mistrust among African Americans. In the past, patients trusted me even if they didn't trust the medical system. But now I began seeing many patients disagreeing with or declining my medical recommendations. Some patients began to see me as an agent of the health-care system instead of as their trusted health advisor and advocate. That dynamic was both surprising and extremely disappointing.

CHAPTER 3

Why Compassion, Empathy, and Respect Matter

I WAS STRUCK BY A LINKEDIN post on November 16, 2021, by Susan David, a Harvard psychologist and author of *Emotional Agility*, in which she defined the differences between sympathy, empathy, and compassion. Here is what she posted:

> Sympathy: I am sorry you are in pain. (Distant)
> Empathy: I can imagine what this pain feels like. (Shared)
> Compassion: You are suffering, and I will do what I can
> to help. (Connected and action-oriented)

Her premise is that a good leader is empathetic, but a great leader is compassionate.

I like her differentiation. We health-care workers need the added dimension of compassion, with its *action* focus. After all, as health-care providers, we *provide* help. Our work is action. But do we always acknowledge that our patients are suffering? Do we really take the time to listen, as well as act?

As I have said, there is no time when a person feels more vulnerable than when they are sick. They may feel betrayed by their body. So many times, I have heard, "I eat well and exercise. How can I possibly have heart disease?" They may feel scared of losing control:

"What do you mean I can't go to work? I will lose my job." And almost everyone feels powerless as they face diagnostic tools and treatments that they don't understand.

This feeling of powerlessness is even more frightening because we live in a world where we could feel more empowered than ever about our health. We have access to information via the internet. We can see our medical records on online health portals. We are often asked to participate in decisions on what tests and treatments we undergo. But here's the truth: Patients are not doctors. They do not have the knowledge, training, or experience to diagnose and treat themselves alone. Even when shared decision-making is involved, many patients may feel that they lack power. That gets worse when their emotions are not acknowledged during the medical process.

Health care should be a humane and emotionally aware field. We shouldn't use the word "care" without caring. Compassion is vitally important. If providers deliver health care objectively, treating people like inanimate objects, the patient naturally feels left out of the process. As a physician, I've learned how much a patient's emotions are interwoven into their physical conditions. We have to address the emotions that go along with our patients' physical illness or condition.

I'd like to share my perspective about this with a story that some of you may remember from the headlines. While it highlights medical racism, it also shows what happens when health-care providers and administrators fail to act in a compassionate, empathetic, and respectful manner.

The Story of Dr. Susan Moore

On December 20, 2020, just weeks after a vaccine was finally authorized for COVID-19, Dr. Susan Moore died of the disease at age fifty-two in Carmel, Indiana. She was a highly respected and popular physician, specializing in general family medicine and geriatric medicine. She left behind her nineteen-year-old son, Henry Muhammed, and two senior parents who suffer from dementia.

I was devastated by her death. I went to high school with Susan, and when I discovered the facts of her medical story, rage overtook my sadness. I was shocked when I learned how she was treated before her death and, afterward, the callous response from the hospital administration. Before being sent home from Indiana University Health North, Susan recorded a scathing video review of her treatment and posted it on her Facebook page, saying, "I put forth, and I maintain, if I was White, I wouldn't have to go through that."

Susan alleged that the doctor treating her had repeatedly ignored her complaints of excruciating pain and wanted to send her home prematurely. The doctor, she explained, told her he felt uncomfortable giving her painkillers and made her feel like a drug addict. "This is how Black people get killed. When you send them home and they don't know how to fight for themselves," Susan posted from her hospital bed. "I had to talk to somebody, maybe the media, to let people know how I'm being treated up in this place."

In a press release responding to her allegations, Indiana University Hospital president and CEO Dennis M. Murphy said that Susan had been a "complex patient" and that during her stay at the IU Health North facility, the nursing staff "may have been intimidated by a knowledgeable patient who was using social media to voice her concerns and critique the care they were delivering." But outside medical professionals and health-care advocates described this account of Susan's hospitalization as a "blame the victim" statement.

Let me tell you a bit about Susan. She was born in Jamaica but, like me, grew up in Michigan. She attended the same high school as me, J.W. Sexton High in Lansing, Michigan, and graduated a year ahead of me. I knew her to be a sweet and funny classmate whom everyone adored. Like me, she earned an engineering degree and then went on to become a doctor. She graduated from the University of Michigan in 2002, received her medical license in Michigan in 2005, and had been a licensed physician in Indiana since 2009.

After testing positive for coronavirus on November 29, she was admitted to the hospital. She detailed her frustration in the video she posted, describing the interactions with a White hospitalist who was assigned to her case. She said her complaints of severe neck pain were disregarded, despite her self-assessment drawn from her years of medical experience. She had to convince her physician she was having trouble breathing before they would order a CT scan. When the scan revealed problems, she was finally given medication to manage her pain, after hours of waiting. She was discharged from that hospital against her wishes, but then the next day she had to take herself to another hospital in the IU Health system, when her temperature spiked to 103 degrees and her blood pressure fell to 80/60. Normal blood pressure is generally 120/80. Susan never came home.

Her son was vocal in the media about his mother's treatment and death. He told *ABC News* that his mother knew her own medical history better than anyone else and should have been seen as a resource for the medical team, not as a source of intimidation for the staff. "I don't understand how knowing your medical history is intimidating to a nurse or hospital staff."

Murray, the hospital president and CEO, was equally vocal. In an initial public statement, Murray said that he was saddened by her death and the loss to her family. He also expressed sadness about the experience she described in the video. He wrote: "It hurt me personally to see a patient reach out via social media because they felt their care was inadequate and their personal needs were not being heard." But, according to Susan's family, neither Murray nor any hospital representatives reached out with an apology.

While Murray promised to assemble a diverse external panel to address potential bias, he defended his staff, saying that he did not believe they had failed on the delivery of care from a technical perspective. He acknowledged that "... we may not have shown the level of compassion and respect we strive for in understanding what matters most to patients" and expressed concern that the "care team did not have the time due to the burden of this pandemic to hear and understand patient concerns and questions."

His statement was met by outrage. Dr. Theresa Chapple, a Black physician and public health advocate from Maryland, wrote on Twitter that after reading Murphy's statement, "I feel gaslit." She told *ABC News*: "It is so utterly ridiculous and also something that Black people have been going through for quite some time in this country, and that includes Black doctors." She pointed out that this occurs when Black people advocate for themselves and their children. "We're dismissed. We're seen as angry, or upset or volatile. 'Intimidating' is a new one that I hadn't heard before reading this." Christie VanHorne, a public health advocate, wrote IU Health complaining that the hospital was "victim-blaming" Susan for the alleged inadequate care she received. "It's honestly a disgrace to the medical profession that they would blame the victim and the nursing team."

More Black medical professionals spoke up in an op-ed piece in the *Washington Post*, pointing out how the COVID-19 epidemic brought out the confirmation of racial inequities in the nation's health-care system. "No matter how well-intentioned our health-care system is, it has not rooted out the false idea of a hierarchy of human valuation based on skin color and the false idea that, if there were such a hierarchy, 'White' people would be at the top," wrote the group, including Dr. Camara Phyllis Jones, a Black adjunct associate professor at Morehouse School of Medicine in Atlanta and former president of the American Public Health Association, with Dr. Aletha Maybank, chief health equity officer at the American Medical Association, Dr. Uché Blackstock, founder and CEO of Advancing Health Equity, and Dr. Joia Crear-Perry, founder and president of the National Birth Equity Collaborative.

Dr. Jones went on to say in an *ABC News* interview, "Dr. Moore knew that she was being mistreated. She knew she was being mistreated because she knew what she was supposed to be getting. So that makes her voice even more powerful when she was calling them out." She pointed out that IU Health needed to acknowledge that systemic racism existed in their system before they could fix the problem. "It's not on one individual nurse to fix themselves or one individual doctor to fix themselves. You have to engage a lot of people, understanding that racism exists, and that it's a problem for the whole system."

Dr. Susan Moore became a hashtag on social media as headlines and articles hit the news throughout the world. Another person had brought awareness to an issue that we all know exists. Countless research studies have found disparate health outcomes for vulnerable populations—racial, ethnic, and religious minorities, individuals living in poverty, individuals with chronic diseases and disabilities, individuals who identify as LGBTQIA, patients who are obese, and more.

But I can assure you that none of that means much to Susan's son and parents. I can assure you that none of that matters to the countless patients who depended on her care. I can assure you that none of that matters to a community that has now had its fabric torn with her death. Because at the end of the day, every life does matter and has meaning. Susan is greatly missed.

How is this an example of the lack of compassion in health care? Compassion means *listening* to the patient as the final source of information on their health. Clearly, Susan was not listened to. Why not? Her advocates are suggesting that it was because she was Black. So we're back to our earlier point that doctors' biases can dehumanize the patient, judging them unworthy of being listened to. Without listening there can be no real compassion.

As a side note, several months later the hospital issued a statement based on the findings from an external review panel of six leading national and local health-care experts to determine whether Dr. Moore received appropriate, compassionate, and evidence-based care, and whether racial bias was present in the delivery and communication of her care. The panel concluded that while the medical management and technical care Dr. Moore received did not contribute to her death, there was a lack of empathy and compassion in the delivery of her care. They also found that in terms of the delivery and communication of her care, cultural competence was not practiced by all providers and several caregivers lacked empathy, compassion, and awareness of implicit racial bias.

While I appreciate that the hospital acknowledged lack of empathy and the need for cultural competency, I was frankly appalled that they claimed that medical management and technical care did not contribute to Susan's untimely death. How can you separate out these factors from her treatment and premature release from the hospital? The hospital CEO described Susan as a "complex patient" and said the nursing staff treating her "may have been intimidated by a knowledgeable patient who was using social media to voice her concerns and critique the care they were delivering." I find it extremely disturbing that a Black woman advocating for herself could be described as "intimidating." I am so incredibly sad that Susan ultimately lost her life as a result.

On Becoming More Empathetic

Obviously, it is clear from Susan's story that we must do better. The health-care industry is working to improve patient experiences, and there has been much research and professional training around empathy and compassion. Most medical schools now require classes on empathy. At Cleveland Clinic Lerner College of Medicine, empathy has been part of their curriculum since the school opened in 2002. I

like this quote from Leonard Calabrese, a doctor of osteopathic medicine who teaches empathy in The Art and Practice of Medicine at the
college: "Empathy is not an option. It is at the core of what we do,
which is why we embrace it... Our organization values empathy,
which is why we teach relationship-centered health-care communication to our medical students."

Researchers and academics are exploring what makes compassion and empathy different in clinical settings compared to the
general world. Cognitive empathy, for instance, is used to describe
a physician's ability to recognize a patient's emotions, reflect those
emotions back to the patient, and consider the emotions when
making care decisions. But there is also affective empathy, when providers internalize the patient's emotions, feeling those emotions
themselves. Traditionally, the focus in health care has been on cognitive empathy, but there is a growing consensus that doctors must
bring both to the table.

While doctors need to detach from their personal feelings to provide care, they also need to recognize that patients want genuine
empathy. Affective empathy can be difficult for health-care providers
because they have been trained that detachment helps them to make
good decisions and prevents a toll on their emotions if they become
too involved. Additionally, affective empathy requires time to connect with patients, a luxury that few physicians have.

But it is worth the time. Research indicates that outcomes could be
improved with more focus on empathy. Multiple studies indicate that
patients who perceive their providers as more empathic can get better
faster and experience less aggressive symptoms. Empathic providers
listen better to patients' needs and engage in shared decision-making.
Patients who feel heard and involved are more compliant with medical
recommendations. In one study, higher scores on the Jefferson Scale
of Patient Perceptions of Physician Empathy were significantly associated with patients' compliance with physicians' recommendations for
preventive tests such as colonoscopies and mammograms.

The Trust Equation

As you can see, compassion, empathy, and respect are crucial to a patient's ability to trust their doctor. While medicine always needs to be evidence-based, that does not mean that doctors can take a cold, scientific approach with their patients. Our interactions must be empathetic. We are not computer programmers or engineers. It's not like going to a mechanic to get your car fixed. Medicine is about human interaction. In health care, we must be able to address how people feel about their condition. We must be able to hear, validate, and address patients' feelings. As a doctor, having your patients trust you is essential.

One useful way of looking at this is by applying the "Trust Equation," originally developed to examine organizational dynamics and often used by marketers in studying their customers.

$$\text{Trust} = \frac{\text{Competency} + \text{Connection}}{\text{Risk}}$$

What this equation says is that customers' trust is based on three factors: competency, connection, and risk. "Competency" means how well a product or service is made and delivered, "connection" means how the customer relates to or engages with the individual or institution developing the product or service, and "risk" means the customer's level of exposure to harm or danger.

Let's take purchasing a quart of milk as an example. The milk needs to be delivered fresh, not spoiled (Competency). You don't need to feel good about the store or individual you purchase from, because that is not a factor in your initial decision-making, where Connection is less important. The chance of being hurt by your milk purchase is very low (Risk). This means that you will probably buy that first quart of milk at just about any store. However, if by chance you do bring home some bad milk, you will probably not return to

that store because they messed up on the one factor that was important to your milk purchase: Competency. And the store has probably
lost any potential Connection to a loyal customer.

When it comes your health, the risk is high, so your decision to see
a doctor is important. To trust your doctor, you need to see them as
competent: You want to make sure they went to a good medical school.
You look at how long they have been in practice. You want to know that
they are up on the latest technology and medical knowledge. You may
check their scores on a doctor-rating site like Healthgrades. You ask for
recommendations from others. And ultimately, you judge their competency by the way they are able to accurately diagnose and treat your
health problems.

Yet for most patients, competency is not enough to build trust. You
also need to feel a connection to your doctor. You want them to remember your name and important facts about you, beyond just your
medical history in your chart. Do they know that you are married and
have children? Do they ask about a recent loss you may have experienced? Do they look you in the eye during an examination, or are they
always typing up their records? Do they ever share things with you that
give you a little window into who they are outside the examining
room? Essentially, do they take the time to build a connection?

I can't tell you how many times I have heard statements like "I knew
he was a good doctor, but he was so abrupt with me," or "I felt she didn't
listen to what I had to say, but I am sure she is good at what she does,"
or "He was like a cold fish. I don't know if I will go back again."

People want to build rapport with their doctor. I think this is particularly critical with primary care doctors, chronic disease specialists,
pediatricians, and obstetricians. These are doctors who are going to be
with you for the long haul, so the Trust Equation has real impact. On
the other hand, if the medical risk is very high in an urgent situation,
I am not sure that connection is such a critical factor in physician selection. For example, if I needed brain surgery, my inclination would
be to go with the surgeon with the highest competency number even

if they were lower on my ability to connect with them. For us doctors who want to build long-term relationships with patients, the connection factor is much more important.

A Non-Doctor's View of Empathy

We doctors can learn a lot from other helping professions. I gained a different perspective on empathy when Kathy interviewed her friend and college roommate, Carol Heinisch, a social worker. Carol is affectionately known among her friends and colleagues as the Queen of Compassion. In addition to being a teacher for genetic counselors, she is the first social worker to work full-time for the Colorado State Public Defender's Office.

She candidly describes what it is like to work with defendants, some of whom are accused of terrible crimes: "As I develop a relationship with that person through the process of working with them, I tend to put what they did, especially in the more horrific cases, on a shelf. What I tell them, and what I believe, is that their action, no matter how horrible it was, doesn't define who they are as a human being. That's my overarching sort of mantra that I give to them. I want them to walk out of the room and feel that someone does not see them as a monster." This reminded me so much of my grandmother, who treated so many vulnerable inmates throughout her lifetime.

Carol practices empathy every day in her work, so how does she look for empathy in her health-care providers? Has she ever felt dismissed? She says she has been fortunate, but has one negative memory: She got a positive home pregnancy test and excitedly went to the doctor for confirmation. "He coldly dismissed me with 'You're not pregnant.' Just like that. I remember feeling totally devastated and knowing he really didn't care." No empathy there.

As an educated practitioner and consumer of professional empathy, Carol's strategy is to carefully screen and select her doctors. "It's a matter of meeting with them and seeing if they give me eye contact. Do I feel like I'm being heard? Is there a sense of lightness, some humor, and a comfort level? I want respect and to be taken seriously. Those factors are really important."

Carol has no hesitation to changing doctors if she does not like the way she is treated. Her reaction falls in line with people who took our Pulse Survey. More than 76 percent said they have changed doctors because they did not like the way a medical professional treated them. It's also important to note that people look at a medical practice as more than a doctor. In fact, when survey respondents were asked who they felt would be most likely to practice empathy when providing a medical treatment, nurses received the highest score at 30 percent, followed by nurse practitioners at 25 percent. Physicians were perceived as most empathetic 20 percent of the time, followed by physician assistants at 11 percent. Clearly, we doctors are not well known for our empathy.

Carol adds three pieces of advice about empathy and how it relates to bias:

1. **Recognize and embrace that fact that you're biased and judgmental.** "If you don't do that, then you're not going to move on, because you're going to be in denial. You're going to try to push it away. You need to say, 'Aha, here comes this judgment, here comes this bias. It is part of me. I don't necessarily like it, but I'm going to put it up on the shelf. I'm going to be here with this person as much as possible.' The people who have the most difficulty are the ones who say they are not judgmental and biased. They're not being realistic about the situation. If they finally see their bias, they end up punishing themselves. They experience internal chaos because they're beating themselves up because they're feeling biased and judgmental, instead of recognizing that it's a natural process."

2. **Allow yourself to feel, and know that there will be tears.**
   She finds this particularly important when working with
   her student genetic counselors, who worry about showing
   emotion in front of their clients. "I say to them that research has shown that patients are very touched when a
   doctor or medical person is so touched by their story that
   they had tears in their eyes. What I tell the students is you
   don't want to be sobbing on the floor so your clients are taking care of you, but it's okay to allow yourself to feel for
   them." That's part of compassion and empathy.

3. **Practice self-care.** "There are lots of things to do to take
   care of yourself. Everyone should have a plan. You can't
   come home night after night and rehash the stories you
   hear in a way that affects you negatively. You have to coun-
   terbalance that with self-care." Here, Carol is advocating for
   self-compassion. Those of us who empathize with others
   all day need to take care of ourselves, too.

We Can Do Better

As Carol practices in social work, we in health care are meant to
create a judgment-free zone. There is no room for bias in our medical decision-making. It is our responsibility to always act with
professionalism, even under the most difficult of circumstances.
Unfortunately, the medical profession has become compassion-
fatigued. Overworked, in debt and underappreciated, we have not
always done our professional best, and so we've lost a lot of respect
over the past few decades. One of the ways we can regain that respect
is by raising our level of professionalism. We can regain respect by
giving respect to our patients.

I first learned about professionalism from Dr. Catherine Lucey,
current vice dean of the University of California at San Francisco's

Medical School and the first person I worked under in a clinical setting. In fact, she's the person who showed me how to take a blood pressure. Dr. Lucey was like a doctor superhero to me. For example, she knew not to take me in the room to shadow her when her patient who was a priest came to the office. There was something sacred in that professional relationship that she wanted to protect.

Dr. Lucey gave the same care to Medicaid patients arriving by city bus as to wealthy businesspeople arriving by limousine. In fact, I think she gave the disadvantaged patients a little more. She treated them with such care, almost like you would a newborn child. In my three years of working with her, I never once heard her bad-mouth a patient. She was always professional, and I am so happy that she was my first example of what a doctor should be.

How many of you remember the television doctor, Dr. Marcus Welby? He was a family practitioner with a kind bedside manner, on a first-name basis with many of his patients. He also made house calls! Remember those? Dr. Welby exemplified compassion and empathy. His patients trusted him. But when I think of how medical care and our medical culture are delivered today, I have to admit that a good number of patients simply do not trust us. We are not Marcus Welby, MD.

The LEAGUE Model

What can we do to put compassion, empathy, and respect back into health care? Here is a simple model that I created for my work with the New York Health Association Symposium on Maternal Mortality in 2018. The acronym is LEAGUE, because I believe we need a league of health-care providers who are up for the challenge of raising the bar on how we deliver care to patients. This is my prescription on how to bring compassion, empathy, and respect into the health-care environment:

Listen more, judge less.

Empathize more, recognize mistrust, and show more compassion.

Avoid making assumptions.

Guard against gut reactions and generalizations about certain groups.

Understand communication styles may differ among different cultures.

Explain more, and don't make assumptions about patients' medical knowledge or literacy.

Let's break it down a bit more:

LISTEN. Listening means really hearing and believing the patient. It's estimated that upwards of 60 percent of patients lie to their doctors. But, according to research, they generally lie to avoid being judged. Yes, we do get the occasional malingerer and need a bit of healthy skepticism when we encounter them. But they are few and far between, and we want to avoid becoming cynical. If you find cynicism creeping in, it may be time to consider another profession. Every time you stop listening, think of Dr. Susan Moore.

Before you speak, make sure you listen enough to understand the patient's issues. Experts say 90 percent of diagnoses can be made from the history alone, but don't just make assumptions from the history. Ask more questions. Avoid interrupting. Ask how the patient feels. And really listen.

EMPATHIZE. I can't overstate how important it is to understand and share the feelings of others. We are not just listening; we are HEARING our patients. Think about how much effort it took for them to get to you. Empathizing involves building a rapport based on mutual respect and sharing of feelings. Let the patient know that you're in this together. You are a team that includes everyone from the providers to the receptionist. Let the patient know that everyone is there to help. Compliment them on the positive things they are doing to take care of their health. Compliments give a boost to confidence and trust.

ASSUMPTIONS. Don't assume you know what they're thinking or assume that you know their plight. For example, some patients feel that doctors think they are asking for pain medications when they are not. Just because a patient is complaining of pain, it doesn't necessarily mean that they are asking for pain meds. Most of the time they just want help of any kind. I'm embarrassed by how often I've heard health providers make assumptions that people are or will become drug addicts. They dismiss the patient's complaints, assuming they are just "drug seeking," rather than taking the time to listen to the patient's whole story. Just think #DrSusanMoore.

It's also easy to make assumptions based on how a patient looks. I have a patient who has severe systemic lupus erythematosus (SLE), the most common type of lupus. (SLE is an autoimmune disease in which the immune system attacks the body's own tissues, causing widespread inflammation and tissue damage in the affected organs.) My patient's case was so severe that she was in such a hyper-coagulable state that she had multiple blood clots while on anticoagulation. She had lupus cerebritis with severe headaches and more symptoms. But when she came to see me, she was perfectly put together, her hair and nails done, and dressed to a T. If I hadn't seen her scans and blood work, I would have thought she was faking. It was tempting to assume, based just on her appearance. But I had to take the time to go beyond the surface.

It's also easy to make assumptions about patients with anxiety, like those who are worried they have cancer when they do not. You keep telling them they are fine and reassuring them that nothing is wrong. You think they don't need help. Your eyes might even roll up in your head when you leave the examination room. Yet, these patients do need your help. They need the right words from you to feel better. Here's a technique I use: I validate them by matching their level of concern. This goes beyond reassurance. Reassurance is given from a distance, while validation is empathy. You can confirm that you really "get it" by responding in kind. Show that you're concerned about their concerns.

PUT A CHECK ON YOUR GUT. Avoid acting on gut reactions that generalize about certain groups. Remember, the brain naturally associates our experiences with past experiences, jumping to generalizations. It takes effort for us to question a knee-jerk assumption that is based on just superficial impressions. What does your gut tell you when you see someone dressed like a gangbanger? Or a patient who is highly anxious or whiny? Or when a Black woman is in labor by herself? Your gut can take you to lots of preconceived assumptions. Don't go with what's in your gut. Look for scientific evidence. Learn more about that individual in front of you.

A story about assumptions: A Black woman comes in complaining of acute and continuing abdominal pain. In her initial evaluation, she was asked if she did any drugs. Being honest, she said she occasionally smoked marijuana. That led to two and a half months of continued agony because the doctors assumed she had cannabinoid hyperemesis syndrome. Black woman? Check. Young? Check. Smokes marijuana? Check. Assumptions: Probably not telling the truth of usage? Check. So, no need for abdominal imaging? Check. The doctors assumed. When this patient finally found a doctor who listened and ordered imaging, she was found to have a large tumor in her stomach. The previous doctors' gut assumptions about her gut, based on stereotypes, prolonged this woman's suffering.

COMMUNICATION. The truth is that sometimes we have bad days. I've had them. Where we're overwhelmed or frustrated, we might even need to fake compassion a bit. Here's a simple go-to line that validates and lets people know you are listening: "I'm so sorry that you're feeling badly. Let's see if we can get you better." Then we get to work. Yet having an occasional "gotta fake it" day is not the same as dismissing people in their most vulnerable time because we don't like the way a patient communicates. Not only do communication styles differ in different cultures but they also differ among individual people.

Take the story of Serena Williams. She's a world-class athlete, superstar, and boss in her personal life. She is also someone highly tuned into her own body. Serena had a history of pulmonary embolisms and was identified as having a coagulation disorder. She had been on blood thinners but was taken off in preparation for a C-section, which made her nervous about the possibility of a blood clot. When she became short of breath immediately after delivery, she was very alarmed and knew something was wrong. Serena got up from her hospital bed and walked out of the room to the nurses' station where she told the nurse something like, "I need a CAT scan and IV heparin, right away."

The nurse told her to go back to her room and that she'd call the doctor. Serena immediately felt dismissed, and this experience caused her great distress. I was disappointed to read that the nurse thought Serena's pain medicine might be making her confused. My disappointment stemmed from the fact that Serena was not being listened to during what could have been a medical emergency. Eventually a CT scan proved her right. She had a pulmonary embolism and several small blood clots had traveled to her lungs. She was put on an anticoagulant heparin drip. Perhaps the nurses could have responded better to the patient's complaint by asking for further information: "Are you having trouble breathing?" or "Do you think you are having another blood clot?"

When communicating with vulnerable patients, we have to use culturally sensitive speech. Become aware of the power of words. For example, most African Americans dislike the term "you people" or using the word "you" in general. In our culture, it's "we," "our," and "us." In fact, in many cultures, when you use the word "you," it is seen

as a way to further accentuate our differences. If a culture is unfamil-
iar to you, do some research. If the only exposure you have to Latinx
people is at work, spend some time making friends in that community. Learn how they communicate.

Some cultures may not want to hear negative news. For example,
there is a great deal of denial with certain disorders among African
Americans. Patients come to me after being diagnosed with diabetes
by other doctors, yet claim they are only borderline diabetic, even if
they are on medication. Many African American patients view their
health through the lens of their emotional health, which means that
if they feel good emotionally, they view themselves as healthy. So
sometimes it's difficult to give bad news to patient about conditions
like diabetes. That's where culturally sensitive communication comes
in. In some cases, it's best to spin the negative news in as positive a
light as possible. "Your blood sugar is super high, but thankfully, we
are confident that we can work together to bring it down." Or "Thankfully, you don't need insulin just yet." Or "If we work together, we may
be able to make this go away."

"Fear Factor"–style coaching has yet to be proven generally effective among African American patients. Trying to scare them with facts
and figures does not work. It is not useful to tell them that they are
three times more likely to have an amputation or blindness with diabetes. But these patients might take negative news better if it comes
in a real story about a real patient, as a cautionary tale to motivate
change for the better: "I once had a patient who had your exact same
problem. Unfortunately, she had a tough time sticking to the program
and she ended up progressing to dialysis. I really think we can prevent that from happening to you if we . . ."

EXPLAIN. I grew up with no health insurance, and although my grandmother was a nurse, many others in my family had low medical
literacy. In medical school, I spent a lot of time re-explaining my at-
tending physician's instructions to African Americans and other

patients because I could tell that they didn't have a clue about what was being said. I'd have to explain it in layman's terms, sometimes using a lot of analogies. It took time, but it helped.

One hard-to-explain area is flu shots. I have experienced a lower acceptance rate for flu shots in my African American patients, even those who are highly educated professionals. One of my patients is a dentist, but she absolutely refuses to get one. So I did a little experiment: For everyone who declined a flu shot, I asked them, "If I had an organic, all-natural pill to take as a substitute for the flu shot, would you take it?" One hundred percent of the people I polled said yes. Then I proceeded to tell them that the main ingredient of the flu shot is organic—the virus is organic. I also told them that I've taken that shot every year for over twenty years. That combination of sharing my own story and understanding where their fear comes from is what did the trick: I had more success in convincing patients to get the flu vaccine. That's the importance of explanation: It's a big part of patient education. Sure, it doesn't work for everyone. There are some folk who are super conspiracy-minded. A family friend thinks the flu shots contain microchips. I explained to him that it would be really hard to disguise a chip in one milliliter of clear fluid. Did I change his mind?

Too often, however, we don't take the time to explain in terms that this particular patient can understand. We simply document that we did our part and that the patient declined treatment. Next time you feel yourself about to write, "patient refused," please take a time-out. For starters, please consider using other language. Using the words "patient refused" paints the patient in a very bad light and can shape the opinions and biases of other health-care providers against them.

The language we use to document our patients matters. It stays in the patient's chart forever, perhaps triggering the biases of providers further down the line. One of my patients has a severe case of systemic sclerosis, in which the blood vessels in her fingers severely constrict, cutting off the blood flow. She was seen at a top hospital, where she complained of pain for months until finally the pain became absolutely excruciating. The doctor there accused her of drug seeking and documented that in her chart, which made her next specialist further doubt the patient's complaints. Dismissed by several doctors, this patient developed gangrene in the distal fingertips and underwent amputation of several of her distal digits. Can you imagine the pain of your fingertips dying off your hand? All because one doctor labeled you with false assumptions and another believed them?

How do you handle patients who decline therapy? First, make sure you are getting *informed* consent, which means that you're not just robo-talking through the fine print and asking the patient to sign on the dotted line. You have to explain the proposed therapy in a way that patient can understand, and then ask if they have any questions. The patient should be able to explain it back to you, including the benefits and risks and consequences of not proceeding. I know this takes more time than we have, but remember that we can use support staff for this. All communication doesn't have to be from the provider.

One of the things we have learned about developing compassion, empathy, and respect between practitioners and patients is that it helps for us to walk in their shoes. There is a joke that doctors make the worst patients, but I have heard many doctors say they developed a new appreciation for what patients go through after they suffered a severe accident or illness themselves. But do patients actually know what doctors and other health-care providers go through, other than the fictionalized version on television and movies? Unfortunately, I believe the answer is no. Let's look further at what it takes to be a doctor.

CHAPTER 4

The Art and Science of Doctoring

I RECENTLY READ A POPULAR advice column where a person wrote in seeking help in overcoming feelings about some of her medical care. For several years, her doctor could not find an answer to her symptoms, even after numerous tests. She believed the doctor thought it was all in her head, even though they never voiced that opinion. She felt dismissed. The writer changed to a new doctor, who found a medication that worked and who recommended lifestyle changes. She now felt better than she had in years. But she still resented the time she had wasted with the first doctor and the loss of quality of life during what she considered her prime years. She was angry and bitter.

I felt for the writer of that letter. Nothing is more frustrating to a patient than not getting a clear diagnosis and treatment that makes them feel better. I understood her pain and the loss she felt from the years where her poor health had prevented her from living the life she wanted. I also know from my own experience that that feeling of being dismissed is common among women.

But I also felt bad for the first doctor. Doctors can't always find the answers. Maybe they were missing something, not asking the right questions, or ordering the wrong tests. Perhaps their frustration made them appear as if they were dismissing her symptoms, while they really were trying to find answers. I don't know the details, but I do know that the fact that the second doctor did find answers does not necessarily reflect on the competency or the attitude of the first doctor.

I was puzzled by the advice columnist's suggestions on how to move on from what she called an "unfair experience." She recommended that the writer use her bitterness to help other people. She recommended writing negative reviews of the first doctor and using social media to tell others about her condition and share the treatment that was working. The advice columnist assumed that the first doctor was incompetent, and it was the writer's duty to warn other potential victims. She also made the risky assumption that the writer could help others if she publicized her diagnosis and treatment on social media. In fact, she could contribute to the epidemic of self-diagnosis-by-social-media, which does not consider each patient's individual differences.

Now let me be clear. I am a proponent of second opinions. I believe strongly that a patient needs answers and should switch doctors if they are not getting what they need. I think doctor-rating sites can be helpful if used properly. What bothered me about this story, however, is the assumption that if a doctor does not get answers, they are instantly and publicly labeled negligent or incompetent.

In the digital world, we believe answers are at our fingertips. People feel empowered that they are able to get so much medical information from Dr. Google. But not all that information is accurate, and even accurate medical information needs to be interpreted and applied by a trained physician. We can also get an unrealistic impression of doctors from the media. Television shows like *House* and *The Good Doctor* portray quirky genius doctors who almost always come up with the right diagnosis and treatment no matter how challenging the circumstances. That's not always the way it is in real life.

We expect to be able to go to the doctor, have tests, and get fixed. The truth is that we doctors are not auto mechanics. Bodies are infinitely more complex than cars. Few people understand how much training we have gone through to be able to diagnose and treat patients. Earlier, I shared the Hippocratic oath, the ethical standard that physicians use as the basis of how they practice medicine. One line that is particularly relevant to our discussion is: *"I will remember that there is art to medicine as well as science, and that warmth, sympathy, and understanding may outweigh the surgeon's knife or the chemist's drug."* This line reminds us that medicine is both an art and science.

On Becoming a Doctor

I feel strongly that we need to educate patients about what it is like to walk in a doctor's shoes. It takes between eleven and fourteen years to become a doctor in the United States. We're talking four years in an undergraduate program, four years of medical school, and then three to seven years as a resident, depending on your specialty.

If all doctors needed to do was go to school to memorize and recall things, becoming a doctor would be really simple. It's not. In fact, it's very complicated. That's why it takes so long to train. It takes years of education, practice, and very long hours—sometimes a hundred hours per week—to get the medical training needed to diagnose and treat. I do not believe there is any other field that requires this much training just to get to entry-level practice in that career.

First, you need an undergraduate degree. I got mine in engineering, but many people study biology, chemistry, physics, or math. Then you take the Medical College Admission Test (MCAT), a qualifying exam required for admission to medical school. While grades, extracurricular activities, essays, and letters of recommendation are all considered on medical school applications, one of the most important criterion is how well you do on the MCAT. In 2021, only 36 percent of people who applied to medical school were admitted. Competition is fiercer than ever.

The good news is that, once you get into medical school, the system is designed to help you graduate as a competent doctor. Your first two years are spent in the classroom, with year one focused on how the body works. You learn every single part of the body—every system, muscle, nerve, artery, vein, and bone—memorizing thousands of parts. In the second year you learn all about diseases. Consider the complexity of just one area, infections: viruses, bacteria, fungi, parasites, and more. Then add in all the other toxins and disorders you have to learn. You are astounded by the sheer volume. After the second year of class training, you take part one of the Boards, the qualifying exam to let you go on to the next level.

During the third and fourth year, you have core required rotations such as primary care, surgery, and OB/GYN. In addition, you choose elective rotations, like plastic surgery. These medical school rotations involve very long hours, eighty to one hundred hours a week. I remember during my surgery rotation, I had to park far across campus in the dark to be on the hospital floor by 4:00 a.m. every day to see patients. At the end of medical school, you take part two of the Boards and then do a residency, where you continue working one hundred hours a week. Different residencies have different training plans and different time requirements, but they are all very intense.

If you are like me, you realize that the biggest challenge is finding time to study while you have to spend so much time in the hospital. You have to see patients but still read, study, and master huge volumes of information for school. Most medical students put their lives on hold, but some do not. I chose to have a child during my second year of medical school, at the advice of a colleague who said it would be easier than later during my residency. Looking back, I don't think I agree. Balancing work, school, and a family were extremely difficult.

On Practicing Medicine

Once you are practicing medicine, first under supervision as a resident and then on your own, all that training, memorizing, and book learning truly does grow into an art and science as you try solving the puzzle of what is causing a patient's distress. The first thing you realize is that diagnosis is not as simple as just plugging in symptoms into a formula and coming out with an answer. Diagnosis depends on the clinician's education and experience with past patients, as well as their application of evidence-based research.

When we say evidence-based, we mean research results that have passed the rigor of a randomized clinical controlled trial. The researchers in that trial have evaluated the effectiveness of an intervention or treatment compared to a placebo and proven scientifically that its outcomes are superior. The results of the new drug or treatment have to be "statistically significant," meaning that your treatment has stronger effects than could happen just by chance. Not all research has such significant results. Not all research studies have tested their treatment on enough people for their results to be meaningful. They don't have real evidence that their treatment works. But those unreliable research studies can still get posted on the internet, spread through social media and street gossip. We medical doctors have to be able to know the difference.

People do Google searches to find out what may be the matter with them or what's recommended to treat a disorder. But they may not understand whether that Google information comes from good scientific research. I hear often, "Oh, I have condition A. I have these symptoms, and my friend had the same symptoms. She took this, she did X, Y, or Z, and it helped her, so I bet it's going to help me." That's a belief not based on scientific evidence; it's just anecdotal. That XYZ "cure" is just one person's story. To believe it is a biased way of thinking. These patients have been swayed by gossip "science." But evidence-based medicine is the exact opposite of bias-based medicine. It has been proven scientifically. New research is coming out all the time, and doctors must continuously keep up with it to be sure to offer the best evidence-based treatments to their patients.

The Challenge of Diagnosis

A symptom can be caused by many different things. Take nausea, for example. Nausea can result from something directly in the stomach like gastritis, an ulcer, a parasite, or a viral or bacterial infection. It can be caused by your gall bladder, liver, or a problem in your small or large intestines. Or maybe you're feeling nauseated by a migraine (with or without a headache) or an issue with your central nervous system, like meningitis. You might be having a problem with your brain or heart. A single symptom like nausea is just the surface sign of many possible problems.

That's why the doctor's getting a medical history and doing a hands-on physical exam are such important parts of the diagnostic process. When we take a history, we glean a lot from what the patient tells us about their past and current health. In medical school we learn a specific methodology for doing histories.

Imagine you come to the doctor's office with a complaint of pain. The doctor will ask about location, quality of the pain, whether it's sharp or dull, its severity on a scale of one to ten, when it started, duration, and if it is constant or intermittent. They will want to know what makes the pain worse and what makes it better. They will ask about other symptoms you're experiencing at the same time. The doctor will go through a whole line of questioning to help sort out and narrow down the list of possible causes. They'll also ask you about illnesses you've had in the past, your lifestyle, and your family's health history. After the doctor gets your in-depth history, you will get a physical exam and possibly blood tests and diagnostic imaging.

All this questioning and diagnostic work gives us first a big and then a more focused picture of what's going on with you. As we gather your information, we consider possible diagnoses and eliminate others. Our goal is to get as exact as possible in our diagnosis and then begin treatment. Once we have confidence that we have identified the problem, we prescribe treatment, see how you react to it, and then reevaluate. If the treatment doesn't work, we might consider an alternative diagnosis and treatment.

Sometimes patients have a group of symptoms that could be caused by many different disorders. Then we have to run tests in order to conduct a process of elimination to help find the correct diagnosis. Some diagnoses are more difficult to determine than others because they have no or very few objective findings. Some of these diagnoses are what we call "diagnoses by exclusion," meaning we have ruled out all the possibilities and settled on a diagnosis by default. Sometimes, doctors refer to this as a "wastepaper basket" diagnosis because we are ruling out or throwing away possibilities. The diagnosis of fibromyalgia is one of those mysterious conditions where its symptoms could be caused by several other diseases. It doesn't have its own distinct symptoms, so we have to diagnose it by elimination. This is a complicated process, calling on the doctor's education, experience, and intelligence.

If diagnosis was simple, then people wouldn't even need to see a doctor. They could type in their symptoms and get a diagnosis from the computer. That day has not come. We still need the doctor. These days, doctors are using computers to great advantage, but the computer hasn't taken over the doctor's job yet. The computer streamlines the doctor's search for the latest research and aids in record-keeping, and the electronic medical record allows medical teams to easily share a patient's current and past information. Telemedicine allows us to "see" patients from a distance; with telemedicine, you can do a great history, though not a physical exam. A good physician can diagnose most conditions. I am not sure I agree to that degree, but I do believe that many conditions can be diagnosed through the history process, especially when it is supplemented with further diagnostic testing. But it takes a trained doctor to analyze that medical history and order the right tests.

Challenges to Treatment

I've never met anyone who wants or likes to take medication. That's understandable, but some patients refuse medication without even listening to the doctor's explanation of why it is needed. Some patients define themselves as a complete "non-medication person." The truth is that nobody wants to take medication, and doctors don't really want to give it.

There is a misconception that doctors *like* to prescribe drugs. Even worse, people believe that doctors are paid by pharmaceutical companies to push drug therapies. This is not true. There is no financial remuneration; doctors are not incentivized to write certain prescriptions. In fact, there are laws and regulations that specifically prohibit doctors to take money for recommending a treatment. False beliefs like this create an unnecessary barrier of mistrust between the doctor and patient.

Why do doctors prescribe medications? Quite simply, we prescribe medication when we have evidence that it will reduce symptoms and prevent further complications from the disease. In some cases, that one little pill could prevent untimely death or the need for more aggressive treatment like open-heart surgery or dialysis.

One of the biggest challenges for doctors is prescribing medication for disorders we call "silent killers," because of their lack of symptoms. A person feels fine, but their blood pressure or blood tests tell the doctor that the person is not fine. Hypertension and diabetes are examples. Since the patient feels fine, they question why they need to take medication. If they decline medication because they don't understand why they need it, this can result in serious but preventable problems.

I get it. You have no problem taking medicine when you feel sick. You want to feel better, so you take what the doctor prescribes. But when you don't feel sick, you might question the need for that pill.

That's why you hear all that talk about "health literacy." Health literacy means getting to know how your body works and how medicine works in your body. You need to know enough about the human body to understand and believe that certain physical conditions lead to others, as when super-high cholesterol leads to clogging of the arteries and possible heart attack or stroke. You might feel fine in spite of your high cholesterol and high blood pressure, but when you learn where those conditions can take you later on, it makes it easier for you to accept medication now. But I'm afraid that, even with education, some people don't believe that their current "fine" condition could get worse untreated. Just like many people didn't believe a pandemic was coming.

Perhaps one problem is how we doctors talk about drugs. We often talk about treatment, not about prevention. "I'm prescribing you X to *treat* your high blood pressure," rather than saying, "I'm prescribing you X to lower your blood pressure to *prevent* a stroke." People love their "nutraceuticals," the vitamins and supplements that are sold as harmless preventatives, even though there is often no science or regulation to support or control their manufacturing or use. People think that, because it's a preventative, it's okay. But there is no proof that they are either harmless or that they work to prevent illness.

Instead of just talking about *treating* high blood pressure, I wonder if doctors would have more cooperation from patients if we talked about a medication *preventing* a heart attack or stroke. If we talked about medically prescribed prevention instead of medically prescribed treatment, people might understand that we are trying to prevent complications and more complicated treatment later on.

Being a Doctor Is Getting Harder

I love medicine. I cannot begin to tell you the joy I feel when I am able to help someone live a longer and healthier life. I consider it an honor to be a physician. But I have to tell you that being a doctor is getting harder and harder, despite all the new diagnostic and treatment tools that should be making it easier and easier. One reason for my discouragement is because the business of medicine is complex. To run an independent practice, a doctor must be not only a top-notch health provider but also a savvy businessperson. I talked earlier about the inadequate insurance reimbursement we get for our services, and that shortage of revenue is a primary reason why it's difficult to keep a medical practice going. The goal is to always to run a medical practice with efficiency, without sacrificing quality. Believe me, it's not easy or for the faint of heart.

But the main reason practicing medicine has become so stressful for both patients and doctors is lack of time. Let me share with you a sampling of quotes from our survey so you hear some examples of the patients' frustration:

> Appointments go fast, they don't remember what happened last time, they are quick to prescribe medications/treatments with little information on effects, they seem to be a little annoyed when asked questions that come from patient research.

> They walk in, ask a couple questions, then diagnose ... vs. digging in to understand. Almost a cookie-cutter response to whatever the issue is.

> I like to know why something is being recommended, and whether it is critical or optional, and what other ways there might be to treat the same condition, and I feel like the doc doesn't have the time to have a discussion—they just assume that whatever they recommend, we will do it rather than want to talk about it.

> Most times I have to stop him going out the door because of time restraints put on him by the hospital protocols that gov-

ern his practice, which is owned by the hospital. He does stop and come back when I protest, though.

Doctor has many appointments with patients scheduled close together and is pressed for time. I believe doctor is working under constraints place on her by the HMO.

I wish I could talk individually with each of these people to explain that we doctors feel the same way. When I was in school, we would do role-playing of doctor-patient conversations, where we would have to explain something to a patient or handle a difficult situation. Most medical schools incorporate patient relationship training, as do courses for nurses, nurse practitioners, and physician assistants. We do know the right and wrong ways to communicate, but when we are always rushing on to the next patient, communication inevitably suffers. And lack of time opens the door for bias and judgment. When we can't take the time to really listen, or to effectively connect with our patients, we are tempted to jump to conclusions based on our biases. It is a big conundrum, but there are ways around it, and it starts with attitude.

Patient First

I am a physician, but I am also an entrepreneur who loves following successful businesses, their marketing strategies, and their offerings. One business I really admire for their name is called Patient First, a chain of urgent care centers in the United States. Isn't that a great name? It also has special meaning to me because the hospital I trained in had a motto: Patient First.

That's where all of our minds need to be: Patient First. We are in the field of health care. It's not about me. It's not about us. It's all about the patients. When we talk about ending bias in health care, we first need to embrace that it's all about the patients. Patient First. If you have a negative bias against a patient who is not "like you," then you are not putting the patient first. That's putting yourself first, because you are judging that patient based on your culture.

Of course, in health care, putting the patient first doesn't mean giving them everything they want. Sometimes what the patient wants is not the best thing for them. This is one of the reasons why in health care, we sometimes have problems with customer ratings. "The customer is always right" style of customer service is not always consistent with good medicine. For example, some patients insist on having an antibiotic for a disease that the doctor knows is viral. Antibiotics are for bacterial infections, not viral ones. We do have to put the patient first, but in some cases that means giving them not exactly what they ask for but what our medical training tells us is best.

What if you want to embrace the Patient First mindset but still find yourself wrestling with your own biases? One of my elder relatives used to say, "I don't know him, but I know his type." At the time, it seemed to me like she was wise in her ability to peg people, but I realize now that was bias. I had to consciously override some of her biases in order to become unbiased myself. It took work and open-mindedness. If you find you have difficulty feeling empathy for certain patients or populations, that should trigger you to work on your attitudes. Therapy or a career coach may be helpful. Your biases may be creeping into the way you work with patients, making them feel dismissed. A dismissed patient is certainly not a Patient First.

CHAPTER 5

A Prescription for Doctors and Patients

I HAVE SHARED WITH YOU some research, personal stories, and patient stories to show you how bias, dismissal, and mistrust on the part of both patients and doctors is so hazardous to health. However, this is not a book about despair and hopelessness. Rather, it is a book about action: What can we all *do* to improve our health and that of those we love?

I would like to give you a taste of what I see as a prescription toward a healthier health-care system. While most of it is aimed at health-care providers, I want to stress that patients also have a significant role and responsibility to take actions in overcoming bias, dismissal, and mistrust.

Rx #1: Be More Relational

As doctors, we have to get back to being *relational* with our patients. That means approaching them in a less fragmented way. That's really tough, because nowadays there's such a shortage of doctors, particularly of primary care physicians. Because of this shortage, practices use a lot of physician extenders, like nurse practitioners and physician assistants. The patient may be seen by the practice frequently, but by a different provider each visit.

So while you may have a doctor who is responsible for a patient's care, that patient may see any of the doctor's affiliates. Even in multiple-doctor practices, patients will rotate through various doctors instead of staying with the one they trust the most and with whom they feel they have a relationship. While this allows doctors to have some semblance of work-life balance, patients end up feeling they are without one person who is their trusted advisor.

Unfortunately, this also means that doctors do not have an opportunity to get to know their patients well. Because of the way the health system is set up, patient care becomes like a factory: Doctors see patient after patient without the time to connect meaningfully with them. It's not like the old days, the *Marcus Welby, MD*, days.

How does being relational connect to bias? Remember the story I told you in the last chapter, about Marianne, the patient with chronic pain? If I knew only her medical condition and not what kind of person she is, I might not have intervened when she was accused of selling her medication and cut from the pain clinic. If I had not had a longtime doctor-patient relationship with her, I might have looked at her with a bias, stereotyping Marianne with the patients I have seen who do misuse and sell drugs.

I see this happen all the time with age, body weight, gender, and race. Because we providers do not have relationships with patients, we don't see them as individuals and so we default to a stereotype. For example, how many times has a patient told me about being discounted because of age? "I knew the doctor was looking at me thinking, 'Well, they're almost eighty. What do they expect?' They don't know that I still work, take care of my house, and travel." The doctor is applying statistical norms, what we expect for an eighty-year-old, to this unique individual who does not fit the norms. If the doctor could take the time to get to know this individual, they would know better than to apply the ageist stereotype.

We have a health-care system that discourages building relationships because of time constraints, cost, and the health-care system structure. In my view, the system's siphoning off of profits and resources from primary care doctors has created a model where doctors must see more and more patients every day. Pushed to increase our volume of patient visits, we are not allowed to focus on quality of care and relationships with patients.

But how can we make health care more relational?

Rx #2: Make Better Use of Primary Doctors

With the changes in managed care, patients can often self-refer to specialists. If they have knee pain, for example, and if their insurance permits, they can make an appointment directly with an orthopedic surgeon or doctor. They don't need a referral from their primary care doctor. This means that they are going to the most expensive provider for something that a primary care doctor could usually handle.

But wait, you say, didn't you just say there is a shortage of primary doctors? Yes, but going directly to a specialist is not always good for the continuity of your health. When you go to different practitioners for different medical issues, it creates a fragmented record. It's not a holistic approach: Nobody is seeing your whole health history as one big picture, so you are left to put the pieces together on your own.

I think insurance companies should consider incentives for patients to go to their primary care doctors for everything. Maybe the incentive is a lower co-pay or premium. Maybe referrals should be required, although that creates more paperwork for doctors. Maybe more patient education is needed. I'm sure incentives can be put into place to send patients back to their primary care doctors for most things. We just need to be open and creative. I do know this: Having one doctor (or health-care team) who gets to know the patients and their conditions well, bodes well for patients' overall experiences and outcomes.

Rx #3: Institute Care Management Reimbursements

A major reason for the lack of a stronger connection between doctors and patients is the way health care is reimbursed. A fragmented reimbursement system leads to a fragmented doctor-patient relationship.

Currently, the only time physicians get paid is when a patient makes an office visit. They have to keep seeing patients to be able to pay the bills. But those office visits are only a part of what patients require. For example, while patients may come in once or twice a year, they call their primaries every time they require a refill, need a letter, or have some other request. When doctors need to communicate test results or other information to a patient, they often have to ask an office worker to call the patient so they can keep seeing other patients in person, for reimbursement. Most of these communication tasks have to be done between visits, and the time spent is not compensated by insurance plans. This puts an enormous time strain on primary care doctors and reduces the amount of personal communication they have with their patients.

Primary care doctors should be reimbursed for care management time, in addition to the reimbursements for in-person patient visits. A more holistic, per-patient payment model would put these doctors at the center of the patient's care. If the practice got fair subsidies to care for patients holistically over the plan year, primary care could actually manage the person's care and take time after hours to call their patients. My own practice participates in innovative programs that set care management fees to help reimburse some of those services that are not compensated under the current system.

Rx #4: Revamp the Affordable Care Act

The Affordable Care Act is a good thing, but it needs serious tweaking. Let's take it from the perspective of patients, doctors, and insurance companies, the three main players.

Patients are frustrated because they believe they pay a lot for their health insurance. Health insurance costs have skyrocketed over the past couple of decades, and consumers perceive doctors and insurance companies to be the beneficiaries.

The problem is that their primary care doctor really does not get much of the money. For example, many patients come in only for a yearly physical, for which the primary care doctor receives about a hundred dollars in reimbursement. It's impossible to run a medical practice on that. In fact, while most doctors agree with the intent of the Affordable Care Act, those who run practices (which are essentially small businesses) have had problems staying in business because of the ACA's low reimbursement rates.

The ACA exacerbated the continuing problem of payments to physicians. For example, it is estimated that up to 20 percent of people who sign up for ACA plans don't pay their premiums and lose their coverage after ninety days. Those patients are not required to pay their doctors for any services they received during that time, and insurance companies only reimburse doctors for visits during the first thirty days. Additionally, there are high administrative overhead and electronic recordkeeping requirements under ACA, which puts an increased unreimbursed burden on that small business.

What about insurance companies? For insurance companies to make money, they depend on the premiums of relatively healthy, low-cost people to help subsidize high-cost patients who run up million-dollar hospital bills. Under the ACA, a patient cannot be charged higher premiums for a preexisting condition. But what if someone is an unrepentant smoker, refuses to get vaccinated, is noncompliant with medication or otherwise continues to make poor health choices that lead to high medical costs? Should that patient's self-imposed preexisting conditions not be considered in setting their insurance rates? Should this person be getting the same insurance coverage at the same price as others? Insurance companies do lose money on some people they insure, but the bottom-line truth is that many insurance companies are still making large profits, or in some cases, exist as nonprofits while paying their insurance executives whopping seven-figure salaries. Of the three players under the ACA, the insurance companies still come out on top.

Rx #5: Create Care Teams and a Medical Home Model

Despite the quality of nurse practitioners and physician assistants, many patients still prefer to be seen by the doctor. Unfortunately, there are not enough doctors to go around. I believe we need to create care teams where one health provider meets with the patient throughout the year for continuity but with full transparency of team support. If we could have a physician assistant or nurse practitioner assigned to a patient for continuity of primary care, we could really work on building ongoing relationships with patients. It would foster trust on the part of the patient and allow the patient to build a more meaningful relationship with their provider. I believe in a "patient-centered medical home" model, not just in name but in how it is paid for and operates. Ideally all patients should feel they have a medical home.

Because of lack of time for provider-patient interaction and failure to provide a medical home, the health-care system has come up with a patchwork of substitutes for real provider-patient interaction, such as online patient portals, population health management tools, and outside care-management services. These are augmented quality-of-care enhancements, but they are no substitute for a practice that can provide full services to its patients at "home," in the practice itself. For example, in my practice we employ four different quality programs from different insurance companies. The insurers interact with the patient in addition to us in an attempt to improve quality. But is this really quality of care? I believe that if the insurers invested directly in the primary care office, we could provide full services ourselves, creating a patient-centered medical home that could be scored on such neglected quality factors as patient communication, empathy, and respect.

Rx #6: Incentivize Doctors Differently

Doctors should be incentivized based on outcomes. If a doctor has disparate outcomes on different factions of their population, they should be held accountable for that disparity or rewarded for smaller health-care gaps. I also think there should be incentives for doctors who take the risk of caring for the most vulnerable patients. If doctors will be penalized for disparate outcomes, they may cherry-pick patients who are more likely to have better outcomes. Doctors who take care of sicker patients should receive higher fees for those patients and more rewards for closing outcome gaps.

Rx #7: Involve Patients in Quality and Incentive Programs

Here's how most quality and incentive programs for physicians work: If an insurance company saves money and the doctor helps it save money and achieves a certain quality score, whatever money is saved gets split between the insurance company and the doctor. This is a grand idea except for one problem. These programs don't adequately incentivize the patient to be fiscally responsible with their health-care dollars. The programs need to be transparent and encourage full team participation, with the patient incentivized in the equation as well.

Here's why. Sometimes patients don't follow what the doctor recommends (big surprise here). The doctor can motivate, encourage, and coach until blue in the face only to have the patient continue their unhealthy lifestyle behaviors. In the current system, the physician is penalized when this happens, along with the insurance companies, as fees are usually higher. What would happen, however, if we gave these patients a portion of their premium back at the end of the year if they stayed healthy and saved money? I believe involving patients in the finances of insurance rates and reimbursement would motivate them to take more responsibility for their health. If they knew that they would receive some financial incentive such as a rebate off their premium or cash back, they might be more inclined to follow their doctor's recommendations. They would have more trust because they would be actively involved in a more transparent system.

Additionally, patients need to be more educated on how their insurance works, and insurance needs to be way less complicated so patients understand what they are getting. For example, patients often say to me, "I pay for my insurance, and I have great insurance." Not surprisingly, when you have a third party paying, you want the most you can get. Sometimes this leads patients to demand medical services just because they think they're "free." But when I tell them that their insurance doesn't cover the procedure and they will have to pay out of pocket, suddenly they don't seem intent on getting the procedure. It's no longer a medical necessity. This is why the patient needs to be an educated consumer of their insurance plan, aware of what it covers, as well as its "perks." The insurance companies often have programs that encourage good health behaviors, such as fitness-center reimbursements and nutrition education programs. These are ways that the patient can participate in their own health care while also being mindful of fiscal limitations in the health-care budget allocated for each patient.

Rx #8: Free Medical School

Almost every doctor who walks out of medical school is leaving with a huge debt. We cannot cut the length of training, because it is absolutely necessary; there is so much to learn. Many new doctors become specialists to clear some of their debt. They know the specialties are much more lucrative than primary care, so we lose many potential primary care doctors to financial necessity.

Because of the shortage, I think primary care doctors should be able to go to medical school for free, or at least have their tuition significantly subsidized. I was able to benefit from a wonderful primary care scholarship that reduced my overall debt, and I'm very, very grateful for that. But I think there should be more tuition subsidies for primary care; it should be viewed as a societal service. Medical students can sign a commitment that they will stay in primary care. Their careers can then be tracked to ensure that they keep that commitment.

Rx #9: Improve the Way We Teach Science

We need to do a better job of teaching science in our schools. Poor science education makes us vulnerable to misinformation, which is creating problems in health care. This is particularly evident now during the pandemic, when we see people chasing after scam remedies and believing false claims about vaccines. We need to develop strategies to counter misinformation and create repercussions for those who apply misinformation to their own and others' health care.

Educating people on the rigor of the scientific process would help fight misinformation. I am very concerned about how little people understand about science and how to be a smart consumer of information. Many people lack the basic understanding of how scientific principles work. They draw conclusions based on anecdote. They see that one set of events precedes another and assume they're seeing a cause and effect. Science doesn't work that way. It uses randomized control trials in the scientific method to prove that there is or is not a true cause-effect relationship. We need to start teaching this way of thinking at the elementary school level.

Many of us have a family member who likes to share their wisdom. Many of us take their word for truth. After all, they pontificate with such confidence. I finally realized that my family's wise woman based her wisdom solely upon her personal experiences. She shares these factoids as if they were gospel, but they are really just what she sees through her own lens. They aren't scientific or absolute principles, but she states them as if they were. That's another reason why we need to arm our kids with a science education—they need to be able to separate fact from opinion.

These nine prescriptions are completely doable. We are not talking about a hopeless situation. The educational and systemic changes I've just suggested can help create a more humane health-care system and more educated patients. What is critical to understand, however, is that attitude is as important as action. If we are able to bring compassion, empathy, and respect into the health-care equation, then we will go a long way in improving the health of all Americans.

PART 2

Too Many Are Dismissed

Prejudice is a great time saver. You can form opinions without having to get the facts.

—E. B. White

CHAPTER 6

Our Biased Brain

W HAT IS BIAS, AND WHERE does it come from? It's complicated, and it's also surrounded by misconceptions of two general types: "You can get rid of bias if you try," or "I'm not biased." My own view of bias changed significantly as I researched this book and talked with experts. I also realized that to truly understand bias I had to look at my own life. What are my biases? How were they formed? How have they affected my decisions? I'll begin this chapter by sharing my personal story in depth.

My Story

I didn't come from a "normal" family with two parents who loved and supported each other. Instead, I was born from a love triangle that was met with stigma against me by the folks of our small town in Michigan. A negative bias came with being a child born under those circumstances. I felt less-than and different. It seemed as if I wasn't supposed to be here. I felt I had to justify my existence by proving my worth to society. I was constantly doing for others, trying to be a "perfect" kid, performing extremely well in school and consoling my mom when she was hurt or depressed. I was the kid whose mother would always say, "Angie never gave me any problems."

When I was five years old, my mother and I moved to Atlanta, where we found lots of successful Black people in the city. I grew up feeling proud of my race, which helped build pride in my identity, especially after the circumstances of my birth. I began to see myself as part of a group, instead of feeling like an outsider. Unfortunately, in Atlanta I became part of a new group not of my own choosing—those people who experience poverty. Poverty brought on new bias against me, and society's judgment excluded me from elite groups like the debutantes and others.

I believe bias also influenced how society perceived my educational potential. My school guidance counselor questioned my ability to handle honors classes. She was surprised when I excelled in science and math. Was her bias because I was disadvantaged, Black, a girl, or living with a single mother? I don't know, but I was determined that nothing would stop me. After struggling to make ends meet for many years, my mother and I moved back to Michigan, where there were programs that supported my ambition. In high school I was accepted into Upward Bound, which I loved. The program is designed to help equalize disadvantaged kids with the advantaged. Upward Bound did not judge us from where we started but instead on what we could be. The CIA Stokes Scholarship, named after the late congressman Louis Stokes, was another great equalizing factor in my life. I am so incredibly grateful for both of these programs and doubt I would be where I am today without them.

After graduating college in engineering, I went to work for the CIA, where I first experienced explicit sexism and racism. It was clear that I was being treated differently as a woman and African American engineer in a White male–dominated field. One male colleague made highly inappropriate comments to me and another female engineer. Others did not share job-critical information because they perceived me as not "one of them." Despite these examples, I did enjoy the mission-critical work that I performed while working there.

After two years, I left the CIA for medical school at George Washington University in Washington, DC. Those first two years in Washington were great, but when I transferred to Indiana University, once again I encountered racial bias. During my residency, for example, favored White students and residents were invited to play golf with the teachers. Of course, I was never invited. When I moved back to Washington I felt included again, especially under the guidance of my medical preceptor and mentor, Dr. Catherine Lucey, who was then the director of the internal residency program at Washington Hospital Center. I was so thrilled and not surprised that her program was one of the most diverse and professional environments I had encountered in years.

My first job as a physician was at a rural health center with a predominantly African American population. I had a fantastic boss and work partners. But when my boss was reassigned, my new supervisor made me feel invisible again. She didn't trust my knowledge and expertise, micromanaging me so much that it felt like harassment. I eventually left that position to start my own practice, where I vowed to value each person, patient, and staff member so everyone would feel important. I continue to uphold this goal every day.

My experiences have taught me that a group or an individual can really make a difference in whether a person feels dismissed or valued. It's one thing to say, "I'm in this group and value it as my preference or my affiliation," but that's quite different from saying, "I belong to this group and other groups are not as valuable as mine." For example, look at the controversy over Black Lives Matter. Why can't people understand that we are not saying that Black lives are more valuable, just that they matter?

I dream of a world where everyone matters, without devaluing any other group. Where we can celebrate our humanity and the intrinsic value of all. Where we can celebrate our differences without making value judgments. Where we appreciate the value of everyone. Yes, that is my dream. So, that is my personal story of living with bias.

Now, what does research tell us about how the brain works on bias? It turns out, *all* our brains are biased.

Brains Use Heuristics

Long ago, our brains developed mental shortcuts known as heuristics to help us make decisions faster. A heuristic works subconsciously to limit the information we have to process. When we need to choose between *A* or *B* and *B* or *C*, heuristics work as formulas that the brain applies to ignore unnecessary information and process the information that the heuristic considers essential. Our brains have learned many different heuristics, but they all serve to save brain-processing time. Without them, we'd be too overwhelmed with data.

One commonly used heuristic is the "availability heuristic." Using this heuristic, the brain tends to give more readily available information more value. For example, we may have information that is recent, often repeated, or has a strong emotion attached to it. The availability heuristic puts that new and familiar information first. You've probably used this heuristic often to make common decisions. You save time by having your brain automatically value certain possibilities more than others.

But we don't often realize that the availability heuristic can also lean us toward biased decisions. For instance, social media platforms use the availability heuristic in refining their algorithms (artificial heuristics like those in our brains) for you based on your location, friends, search history, and interests, so as to feed you just the information that reaffirms what you already believe. Our attachment to and certainty of our worldview are reinforced to the point where we devalue any beliefs outside our own. By overvaluing information just based on how available it is to our own minds, we can build erroneous perceptions and stereotypes of other groups.

Why would such a heuristic exist if it so often leads to erroneous perceptions? How does it help our decision-making? As noted in *The Handbook of Evolutionary Psychology*, we should not assume that this bias-making flaw "in the design of the mind," has always been a flaw. The heuristic may have been useful as early human beings evolved. When the hunter-gatherer met someone who looked different, it may have been wise to fear them. Fearing outsiders may have helped to keep their people safe in those days.

As humans flourished and spread across the globe, our world changed from that of our hunter-gatherer past. We no longer needed to see every outsider as a potential threat. The fear of outsiders, however, remained. Some people found fear to be a tool to gain power. It helped those with means to assume supremacy over those without. They justified their supremacy by a fear of others' differences. This is how those in power have justified treating people of color, Indigenous populations, and women with robbery, slavery, and murder throughout history.

I was startled to learn how early heuristics and bias can start in an individual. I had thought that bias would develop as you grew older, along with adult cognitive understanding and the overload of information that comes with time. I was incorrect. In one study, infants were shown faces of their own race and of other races paired with happy or sad music. The nine-month-old infants showed a preference for looking at faces of their own race paired with happy music, and other races paired with sad music. They were not only already starting to show an affinity for their own race but also a discomfort with a different one.

In another study, four-year-old boys and girls were shown images of Black and White children. Even though the group included both races, the children showed a strong pro-White bias, consistently favoring the images of White boys and girls over the image of Black children. All the children showed the same level of racial bias. I found it heartbreaking that at such a young age Black children have already become biased against themselves.

This is how society is telling children to feel about themselves. In a study published in *Social Cognition*, it was shown that racial biases directed toward Black adults are also applied to young Black children. Our children are taught these lessons far too young. Negative stereotyping and prejudice against Black faces occur no matter what the age.

Explicit vs. Implicit Bias

Bias is defined not only by psychologists, philosophers, and researchers. Government has also gotten into the bias-definition business. According to the U.S. Department of Justice, "Explicit bias is the traditional conceptualization of bias. With explicit bias, individuals are aware of their prejudices and attitudes toward certain groups. Positive or negative preferences for a particular group are conscious. Overt racism and racist comments are examples of explicit bias."

Today, fewer people overtly subscribe to biased isms such as racism, sexism, classism, ageism, heterosexism, or tokenism. Some people have changed their thinking once they acknowledged that bias harms our society. Others hide their biases to avoid the consequences they might suffer from being seen as overtly racist or misogynist.

Additionally, our political systems have installed legal safeguards meant to prevent or punish behavior and language that practice explicit bias. This has happened at both the federal and state levels. For example, federal antidiscrimination laws protect employees from being fired based on race, gender, age, religion or disability, and some laws prohibit discrimination based on sexual orientation. As for another "outsider" group, despite the prevalence of larger people these days, employment bias based on body type is not prohibited. Weight is not protected from discrimination under federal law. This means that most employers can legally fire or take other negative actions against employees for being overweight. That form of explicit bias is still legal.

While overt or explicit bias is less accepted in America today, bias is still heavily ingrained in our culture, legal system, languages, and traditions. These inbred legacies of bias are called implicit bias. Also known as implicit social cognition, implicit bias is the unconscious attitudes and stereotypes that affect our understanding, perceptions, actions, and decisions.

Unfortunately, it is nearly impossible for us to avoid having implicit bias. A study published in the *Journal of Personality and Social Psychology* found that implicit preferences, once formed (and remember, we start forming those in reference to race at nine months old), are insensitive to modification. That means they are difficult to change. Similar findings published in 2010 in *Social Psychology* showed that exposing racially biased people to "admirable" members of the stereotyped race shifted their race bias reliably, but only weakly.

The bottom line is that everyone has implicit bias. We can't avoid having it, but it's when we don't recognize it in ourselves and then make decisions based on stereotypes that we get in trouble as a society. It becomes a particular problem when our actions are driven by biased assumptions about race, body type, age, or gender. Nobody is without bias, explicit or implicit. Health-care providers are no different, but, because of our power position, the effects of our biases can be profound.

Bias in Health Care

Academic and clinical researchers have studied health care and bias from almost every angle of inquiry: What is it, how does it affect different groups, how does it affect the medical team, what are the consequences for specific diseases, does antibias training work, and a host of other questions. Type "bias in health care" into Google

Scholar and you will get more than four million results. I'd like to share a few studies that got me thinking, and I hope they do the same for you.

A comprehensive review published in the *American Journal of Public Health* in 2015 laid bare a health-care system plagued by implicit bias, leading to significant disparities in access to health care, quality of care, and morbidity. Using data extracted from fifteen studies, this article found that the level of implicit bias among health-care professionals mirrored that of society at large. The review found that bias led to poorer quality of care, more barriers against accessing care, and a general lack of satisfaction with health-care interactions. According to the review, the color of your skin also affects your likelihood to survive birth. The infant mortality rate was shown to be higher for people of color (except for Asians) than White people. Black people pay a "mortality penalty" in our country. That's the difference between the lowest mortality rate (that of the White and Asian babies) and the Black mortality rate. Black newborns die at three times the rate of White newborns. I'm not trying to argue that White physicians don't care about Black babies, but it is apparent by the numbers alone that implicit bias plays a large part in deciding who lives or dies.

In the *Journal of General Internal Medicine*, a study proposed that doctors take the perspective of patients, focusing on the individual patient rather than on any preconceptions the doctor might have about the patient's social group. The authors conclude that, if we want to decrease the effects of implicit bias on medical care, all physicians need to acknowledge their susceptibility to implicit bias, practice deliberate perspective-taking and individuation of their view of patients. Furthermore, an increase in the number of Black physicians could reduce health-care disparities, as they have been shown to exhibit less implicit racial bias.

I was puzzled by a 2014 survey of medical students that found that 77 percent accepted that unconscious bias might affect their clinical decisions or behaviors. This is well above the percentage of the general population that believe they are affected by implicit bias, so kudos to those medical students for that. But if so many health-care professionals are "woke" about their own capacity to exhibit implicit bias, why do such health disparities still exist?

Now let's look at bias against the health-care system. That's right, even patients sometimes show bias against those who treat them. Two types of bias are confirmation bias and blame bias. Let's first look at confirmation bias. We've all used these words: "I knew it." If we steadfastly believe something, we might ignore all evidence to the contrary and amplify "evidence" that supports our beliefs. Confirmation bias against health-care providers runs particularly high in certain groups. They mistrust us even beyond the baseline level of mistrust found in the general population. The group I am most familiar with, because of my own background and medical practice's population, is African Americans.

One historical reason why African Americans bring mistrust and confirmation bias to their health-care encounters is the Tuskegee experiment. The memory of the evil of that experiment is ingrained in the collective consciousness of most African Americans. Even though the experiment is long over, I was not surprised when a young Black man who works with my co-author, Kathy, referenced Tuskegee as one of the reasons why he was not getting the COVID vaccine. Though highly intelligent and well read, he was still suspicious of the vaccine because he knew the history of deceptive and harmful medical research on Black people. He said it in one word: "Tuskegee."

Here's a recap of the Tuskegee experiment. The United States Public Health Service promised free medical care to African American men from 1932 to 1972. But what the government really wanted to observe was the natural history of untreated syphilis. Instead of providing real treatment, in this experimental atrocity on Black men, the researchers disguised placebos, ineffective methods, and diagnostic procedures as "treatment." The men who had syphilis were never informed of their diagnosis, despite the risk of infecting others. They were never told that the disease could lead to blindness, deafness, brain damage, heart disease, and bone deterioration, and they were never offered a cure. Please note that this experiment went on for forty years. Forty years!

Black people remembered, but apparently, White America did not. It was not until 1997 that President Bill Clinton issued a formal apology on behalf of the United States government: "What was done cannot be undone, but we can end the silence. We can stop turning our heads away. We can look at you in the eye, and finally say, on behalf of the American people, what the United States government did was shameful, and I am sorry." But Bill Clinton's apology was clearly not enough for the many Black people who still mistrust the medical system. Black people also remember Henrietta Lacks, the African American woman whose cervical cancer cells were kept for research at Johns Hopkins without her informed consent or permission. And these stories are just the tip of the iceberg. We remember and compound them with our own confirmation bias. Every time we hear a dubious story about medicine, we say, "I knew it."

Blame bias differs from confirmation bias in that it blames an individual, not their group, environment, circumstances, genetics, or other factors outside of that individual's control. Blame bias is rapidly increasing, even among doctors. In health care, it has been amplified by patients' belief that we can prevent illness if we simply live a "clean" lifestyle. If you exercise and don't smoke, you will not get lung cancer. If you eat a plant-based diet, you will not have heart disease. If you eliminate sugar, you will avoid diabetes. The truth is that lifestyle factors like diet, exercise, sleep, and stress reduction can help prevent disease. Minimizing those risk factors is good for your health. But, and it is a very big BUT, people get sick all of the time for no reason. Life (and death) happens. We can't always blame lifestyle.

The uneven power dynamic between health-care providers and patients can bring on blame bias at a time when people are in their most vulnerable state: in pain, sharing personal information, and often literally naked. They walk into a doctor's office or hospital and feel judged and blamed that they have brought health problems upon themselves. And the truth is that it really happens way too often.

This fear of being blamed came out strongly in the patients who answered our Pulse Survey, for many things: drug seeking, withholding information from the provider, and for the doctor's assumptions about their lifestyle.

> A psychiatrist didn't believe I had ADHD and refused to treat me. I had been diagnosed by a different doctor five years prior. The new psychiatrist thought that my grades had been too high for me to have had ADHD and he accused me of drug seeking.

> Two years ago, I had a sore throat. I thought it was a cold and just did supportive care. My sore throat got worse. I went to the NP (white woman). She examined me, did a rapid strep test that came back negative, and did throat cultures. [She told] me that I was being a baby. Then proceeded to tell me I was overweight and needed to lose weight. I already know that, and that is not why I was there to see her. I was feeling really bad and didn't have the energy to engage with her. She sent me home with instructions to gargle with salt water. A couple of days later, she called to confirm her assumption that I was being a baby, the cultures were negative. Two days later, on Christmas Eve, I was having difficulty and my husband made me go to the ER. I was admitted to the hospital and spent four days, inpatient with an esophageal abscess. The bacteria that caused the abscess is not normally seen in adults. But the NP was so convinced my pain was not real, she failed to investigate further. I felt like she thought I was

looking for drugs or just not in tune with what was going on with my body.

While caring for [an] elderly family member, [I] had chest pain & elevated blood pressure. Was impossible to get through to a Dr. that was in my practice, and the front desk staff refused to have the doctor call me back. Made an appointment to see the practice's cardiologist and he told me, without asking for any background, that elevated blood pressure was due to not exercising (he hadn't asked if I did or not), that pre-menopausal women did not have heart attacks, and that I needed to stop drinking/eating PepsiCo products (he had not asked what my normal diet was like). It was frustrating! I went to see a female cardiologist in another practice, who took the time to get a full history and what was going on in my life. Her diagnosis was situational hypertension and she had good practical advice, which was super helpful.

In undergrad, I was prescribed a medication for an infection, and [soon] after taking the medicine, I began to feel warm and itchy all over my body. I went back to the medical provider (a white female) who prescribed the medication and shared my symptoms, but because she couldn't see any irritation on my (dark) skin, she dismissed my concerns. I couldn't bear the itching, and the next day began scratching and suffered increased irritation, redness, and swelling. I went back again, and at that time, when she could finally see the manifestation of what I was previously describing, she determined I was having an allergic reaction to the medication. She also told me that I should have been clearer about the symptoms during my previous visit—to which I responded,

"I told you exactly what I was experiencing, and you didn't believe me." I changed providers after that experience.

Jarvis: A Story of Blame Bias

One person whose story really gave me a window into the power of blame bias, and particularly how it relates to medical racism, is my cousin Jarvis DeBerry. Jarvis is new in my life, a previously unknown cousin from my father's side of the family. His story is powerful, since he is a Black man with kidney disease. An articulate and well-known columnist who formerly wrote for the *Times-Picayune* in New Orleans and is now an opinions editor at MSNBC.com, Jarvis has written powerful pieces about his own disease and treatment, medical racism, maternal morbidity, and health-care disparities, particularly concerning COVID.

When he was in his twenties, he was diagnosed with high blood pressure, which is often associated with kidney disease. Years later, his lab work indicated his kidneys were not functioning properly. He was diagnosed with focal segmental glomerular sclerosis, or FSGS, a condition that causes severe damage to the kidneys. He eventually received a kidney transplant.

In one powerful column, he reflected on what he described as one of his most deeply rooted fears: being dismissed, disrespected, and disregarded by others who assumed he had brought the disease upon himself. "Nobody ever wagged a finger or looked down their nose at me or tried to make me feel small for having kidneys that were failing. But I still walked around with the fear of being judged. I still tried to dress a certain way, lest a casual appearance give the impression that I'd been casual about my health."

I had an in-depth conversation with Jarvis that was heartfelt and insightful. I'd like to share some of his perspectives from his ten years of diagnosis and treatment. First, he told me that it was important for him to walk into a doctor's office presenting the perfect image: He would dress up and speak in a manner to present himself as sophisticated, knowledgeable, and respectable. His compensatory strategy was based on his previous experience of the bias directed at him as a Black man in our society.

"I do this in all kinds of new situations. In the medical field, the stakes are higher, so it is even more important. You don't want your doctors to 'write you off' and not take you seriously. I was worried about what they would think of me. Are they blaming me?"

He said he has been treated well by his medical team, with a few exceptions. One surgeon, who needed to do a procedure so Jarvis could take dialysis at home, was cold to him. Jarvis didn't know if this was because he was just a cold person or had a prejudice against Black people. Interacting with multiple health-care providers, Jarvis developed a rapport with many members of his team. Some touched him deeply. Years after he'd first seen his original nephrologist, the doctor ran into him at the hospital and embraced him. "I had never been embraced by a physician before. I was almost taken aback because I wasn't expecting that kind of affection."

Primary physicians played an important role in his health. His first primary was concerned about his high blood pressure at age twenty-two, and years later referred him to a specialist. "We developed a relationship like I was one of her sons. I felt a real concern for my well-being." He feels similarly about his current primary doctor. "She walked into [the] room and was so warm, asking all these questions that were specific to me. Just her asking and remembering that I had a daughter put me at ease."

All his life Jarvis has worked at disproving racial stereotypes, so he was particularly chagrined at getting a diagnosis of high blood pressure as a Black man. Black men are at the highest risk for kidney disease from high blood pressure. Initially he thought he would literally outrun the hypertension by training for a marathon, but his blood pressure remained high. He needed to go on medication.

"I felt defeated by this diagnosis. What had I done wrong?" At one point, he even wondered if eating too much fried chicken had brought on the high blood pressure. Then he finally stopped blaming himself and no longer tried to figure out why this had happened to him even though he took very good care of his health. "I realized it wasn't anything I did. It took me a minute to get there and realize the 'why' doesn't matter. I let go of the unfairness of it all."

Jarvis then quoted me a passage from the New Testament in which Jesus says: "He makes his sun rise on the evil and on the good and sends rain on the just and on the unjust." I cannot begin to tell you how much this moved me. It is one of my favorite passages and has guided me through so much personal and professional trauma. Knowing that as family we both shared this belief that good and bad things happen no matter what made me feel so connected to him.

Jarvis had lived in fear of being blamed for his own illness, but in the end has found peace in the knowledge that sometimes no one is to blame.

Addressing Bias

At this point, you understand that bias is not a dirty word. It is part of our life. It originates from our brains' need to take a shortcut in coming to conclusions. Unfortunately, it can reinforce—often incorrectly—our affinity for and certainty of our own worldview, so much that we no longer value any beliefs outside our own. It happened to me as a child: People believed my mother was living wrongly, so I was made an outcast. Schools made assumptions about my ability to learn based on my skin color and poverty. Bias profoundly influenced my own access to proper health care as a child and teenager. Later on in my life, a doctor's bias led to the death of my infant son.

The question is what can health-care providers do to diminish the effects of bias? For confirmation bias, it starts with our building trust in our engagements with vulnerable populations and, hopefully, improving their health. We have to get in tune with who they are and what they are saying to us. We have to earn back their trust. Yes, I understand that we are over-regulated, the insurance hassles are a drag, and, quite honestly, taking care of patients can be emotionally draining work. But we were chosen to be doctors because we are able to do this. We are able to do better!

How we talk to our patients goes a long way in reducing blame bias. Simply starting off an examination with a statement like "Let me see what I can do to help you get better," reassures a patient that you are there for them, not judging them. It is also important how we react to aspects of their lifestyles that we know are not good for them. I have many patients who smoke, don't exercise, or are significantly overweight. I know that they know their health would improve if they made changes. My harassing them would just make them feel worse. It would not change their behavior.

Take smoking, for example. I do not believe that there is one person in America who doesn't know that smoking leads to all sorts of health problems. Does it pain me to see my patients still smoking? Absolutely. But I tread very lightly by saying things like, "If you are not going to stop smoking, let's see what we can do to help you cut down on the amount," or "You've told me this isn't a good time for you to stop smoking because of what's going on in your life. Let's put it on hold and readdress it in a couple of months." That kind of dialogue can encourage patients to let us help them in the long run.

It's very difficult for a doctor when a patient is noncompliant with a treatment. Some doctors will actually "divorce" a patient from their practice if they don't do what they are asked to do. There are pro and con arguments about this, but what I do know is that before any physician divorces a patient, they need to really understand where the noncompliance comes from. They cannot make assumptions from their own biases against that patient's social group.

Again, our Pulse Survey provided some interesting perspectives on why people do not do what their doctor asks.

> I requested treatment plan NOT to include chemo, doc refused, [and] I was eventually fired as a patient because he stated I did not comprehend the severity of my disease. New oncologist, different plan, twelve years later and I am still in remission.

> My doctor has already decided my treatment protocol, when I share concerns, they don't discuss other options, he continues to reaffirm his position. DOES NOT LISTEN. One-size-fits-all approach.

> The doctor tried to force me to take a hypertension medication, although I did not have high blood pressure. She wanted to write the prescription, because of what she was reading in medical journals about hypertension and Blacks.

> If I do not follow a doctor's treatment instructions, the reason most often is because I cannot afford to.

It has been personally and professionally challenging for me to acknowledge my bias against patients who will not get vaccinated. At the height of the vaccination push, I was even considering not allowing unvaccinated patients to come to my office, because I really wanted to try to convince people to get vaccinated. This is a really tough one, particularly when you are aware of blame bias.

I was and am legitimately concerned about the risk to my staff and other patients. Should I be caring for someone who could have a highly contagious and deadly disease, when they're not doing what they're supposed to do, like wearing a mask or getting vaccinated? Is this blame bias? Doesn't our ethical standard say we need to be self-less and care for all people even if they pose a risk to our health? But in this case, they are making the decision to not do the right thing. What is my responsibility as a doctor? This one keeps me up at night. I don't have a solution. What I do know is that my being aware of my bias and constantly questioning it are important in helping me make the right decisions.

There is not just one form of bias, and there is not just one way to find answers. We do have to recognize how dismissal and cultural bias work against different groups based on race, body type, gender, age, and other factors. By diving deeper into the specific struggle of each group, we will be able to find solutions.

CHAPTER 7

The Threat from Medical Racism

WHEN I WAS REVIEWING THE research on medical racism, a colleague asked me if I was surprised by anything. I realized that no specific study shocked me. Rather, I was stunned by the *volume* of valid research that *directly linked health outcomes to racism.*

Medical racism, defined as systemic racism against people of color within the medical system, has been extensively observed and measured. For years, researchers have been churning out studies of bias in health-care workers, racial inequities in health coverage, and disparity in health outcomes. I found hundreds of studies, primarily relating to African Americans, that confirmed that *medical racism is real.* When a study can objectively quantify that health outcomes are different among different populations, we have concrete evidence: Medical racism exists.

As a doctor and an African American, I was validated as I saw the evidence accumulate. Medical racism was not just something in my head, but something that can be measured and tracked. Research shows us the cause-effect relationships between systemic racism and health outcomes, for which we can then hold the system accountable. That understanding gives me hope. If we care enough to make changes, there are actions we can take. Of course, it is disappointing that we *don't yet have major initiatives in place to address medical racism.*

My colleague asked me if this made me angry. I thought a moment and said no, I was not angry, just tired and frustrated.

For a Black person in America, racism is inescapable but complicated. Since it is often covert, we sometimes doubt our own sense that racism is at work. Am I being treated this way because of my skin color? Is it because I am a woman? Was the person simply having a bad day? Am I having a bad day after other microaggressions and feeling sensitive? Bias, prejudice, and racism can seem subjective. What I can tell you is that most Black people usually assume we are not being treated equally because of the color of our skin. The individual stories abound along with the scientific research.

I never underestimate the power of a story. The world was awakened by the story of George Floyd's murder and his words, "I can't breathe." In that light, I want to share four stories of medical racism. These stories come from my patients and consultations, all African American women. They will show you the individual human cost of bias.

The Story of Ms. Brown

Ms. Brown had an abnormal EKG, so I sent her to her cardiologist for a stress test. At a follow-up visit, I asked if she had seen the cardiologist. She told me her cardiologist had told her she didn't need the stress test. I sent her back again with firm instructions to tell her cardiologist that she did need a stress test: Her EKG was abnormal and had changed from a previous recording. She visited the cardiologist and again came back to me with "She said I didn't need it."

I requested a copy of the consult notes from the cardiologist. These are some of the things that the cardiologist put in my patient's chart:

> Chief complaint: Follow-up anomalous coronary artery, un-
> mitigated cardiovascular risk factors.

Summary: Patient has been noncompliant on medications intermittently. She is at extremely high risk for stroke, MI [heart attack], and death. On dietary review, still eating daily sausage, bacon, ham, fried foods, and cheese despite my extensive counseling. Not exercising, she has no time for herself, she takes care of her sick family. Eating out every weekend. LDL has increased to 136 on 20 mg of atorvastatin. Has gained a tremendous amount of weight. I referred her to the weight management program, but she told me they were 'too White' for her. Extensive dietary and exercise counseling was provided. She always appears motivated in the office when I talk to her but does not carry through. She wants me to carry out cardiac testing. I have advised that in the presence of such poor, unmitigated cardiac risk factors, it is pointless to carry out a stress test. Very frustrating visit.

I was appalled by the doctor's assessment. Ms. Brown is compliant with my recommendations and does take her medication. She has had side effects from some of the drugs, so we have adjusted them. She does not eat sausage, bacon, and ham daily. In the five years I have seen her, her weight has fluctuated from 177 to 195, then down to 188, an eleven-pound gain over five years. I would not call that "a tremendous amount of weight."

I immediately sent her to another cardiologist, an African American. She called me after the visit, very concerned. "This patient needs a stress test like *yesterday*. I'm so glad you sent her."

The first cardiologist's lack of empathy and respect for this patient could have led to her death had we not intervened. Do I believe this was an incident of medical racism? Absolutely. Ms. Brown was dismissed by a biased doctor who saw what she wanted to see. Would she have treated a non-Black patient in the same way? I don't think so.

The Story of Keisha

A friend's daughter was having ongoing abdominal pain and had seen multiple doctors. The pain seemed to worsen with her menstrual cycle but was present most of the time. At one point, Keisha's pain was so severe that she decided to go to the emergency room to be evaluated.

During her interview process at the ER, she was asked if she drank or smoked. She answered the question honestly, saying she occasionally smoked marijuana. At that point, it seemed to Keisha that the doctors felt they had found their answer. They told her weed smoking had caused cannabinoid hyperemesis syndrome, which was causing her abdominal pain and nausea. She was sent home.

Keisha was appalled, especially since she rarely smoked. She felt the doctor tried to pigeonhole her as a drug user. Three weeks later, she was back in the emergency room with the same intense pain. But this time she received an abdominal CT scan, revealing a large tumor in her small intestine. After surgical removal of the tumor, Keisha then had a bleeding complication. Her hemoglobin was very low at 6.3 (normal 11.3–15), but no one at the hospital seemed to feel the urgent need for a blood transfusion.

Her mother asked me to intervene. I spoke with the doctor in charge of her care, only to find out he was a resident and that the attending/lead physician was not even in the building. I told the resident that I was concerned for Keisha's safety. I believe that as an African American woman, her care had been subpar, and that the urgency of her condition was being neglected. I was not polite when speaking with the resident. In fact, I raised my voice during this conversation. I realized that having lost my son under similar circumstances made me angry and less polite in my conversation with this resident who was dismissing my friend's daughter. Immediately after our conversation, Kiesha was transferred to the ICU for closer monitoring. Thankfully, she survived and is doing well.

As in many minority patients' stories, it's hard to know if Keisha was misdiagnosed and then mistreated because of her gender, age, or skin color. The hospital had missed the correct diagnosis at the first ER visit because their bias focused on her marijuana smoking, even though that was very infrequent. Then after her surgery they displayed no urgency when Keisha needed an immediate blood transfusion. Would she have died if her mother did not know an African American woman doctor and asked me to intervene? I don't know, but I am glad I was there.

The Story of Makala

We were seeing an African American woman for routine care, but when my physician assistant entered the examining room they found Makala lethargic and slurring her speech. We immediately called 911. By the time the EMS arrived, she was more alert, but still complained of difficulty walking and numbness in her face. We were concerned about a possible stroke.

The EMS workers asked her questions and took a few vital signs, including her blood sugar. Her blood sugar was 58, which was low, but not low enough to explain her symptoms. The EMT asked us for snacks or juice to raise the blood sugar, but we refused, knowing that in the case of a stroke, the patient should be kept fasting.

The EMTs seemed to be working her up as if they were trying to diagnose Makala themselves, instead of sending her to the hospital right away. We knew that there is a narrow window for effective stroke treatment. When I questioned what was taking so long, they replied that they had to follow their protocol and make sure she was stable. After another twenty minutes, I insisted, "She needs to go to the hospital NOW." They replied, "We can't take anyone who does not want to go." "She WANTS to go!" I exclaimed, as Makala nodded her head yes and said in slurred speech, "I need to go to the hospital!"

In total, those EMTs spent fifty-three minutes in our office before finally taking Makala to the hospital. That is well beyond the time window for standard of care for a possible stroke. I found out later that one of our staff had shared Makala's medical history with the EMS responders. She had a history of IV drug use far in the past, but she had been clean for decades and exhibited no signs of any relapse.

To this day, I wonder if it was the color of her skin or history of drug use that affected her care the most. For Black women, the overlap of race and gender makes for two strikes against them in the eyes of some medical providers. By the way, Makala had indeed suffered a stroke. That fifty-three-minute delay could have cost her life, and definitely did impede her recovery.

The Story of Ms. Edgar

Ms. Edgar has multiple sclerosis and uses a wheelchair. She often calls our office for her medical needs instead of coming in. She also has complete bladder incontinence and smells strongly of urine, so has difficulty finding willing and affordable transportation.

Because of her transportation situation, she had missed several appointments with an MS specialist. They divorced her from their practice, but I called to ask if they would take her back on. They gave her another chance but said that if she missed another appointment she would be banned forever. Ms. Edgar made that appointment but missed the following one. She couldn't afford transportation. As a further blow against her, this practice includes many other specialists who could have helped her, but, unfortunately, once a patient is divorced from one doctor in the practice, they are banned from all. The only other practice I would consider is even farther away from her home. So currently she not receiving any specialized treatment for her multiple sclerosis.

A home care physical therapist called me to report on her home setup, which had stairs. She lives with an ill brother, and neither of them could manage the stairs safely. Both of them have had falls on those stairs. The siblings are doing their best to keep each other alive. We contacted the local Office on Aging to get Ms. Edgar some help at home, and we are working on a home care model for her. But it is likely that her health will continue to deteriorate. She can't get to a doctor, pay for medicine, or get treatment for her multiple sclerosis.

I believe that if Ms. Edgar dies, it will not be simply from her disease; she will die because she is Black and living in poverty. She is far downstream in the flow of the social determinants of health: From racism upstream flow economic inequity, poverty, substandard housing, inadequate transportation, and lack of access to health care.

Others Speak Out

In addition to stories from my patients, medical racism was a dominant theme that emerged from our Pulse Survey. Forty-six percent of the people who answered the survey believed they had been treated differently by a health provider because of either their race or ethnicity. Thirty percent said they would select a doctor who was the same race. Their reasons for this decision varied. Thirty-seven percent believed a doctor of the same race would understand them better; 24 percent felt they would be more comfortable with them; and 19 percent said the same-race doctor would listen better.

In their anecdotal comments, our survey respondents often mentioned race as the reason they believed they were misdiagnosed, given poor treatment, or treated poorly:

> I've been under-medicated; treated like I don't have [an] education; and dismissed by my White physicians many times. It's been very difficult.

In my twenties, the doctor looked at my skin and assumed I had AIDS. They brought some medical students in the room (about five) without asking me, to show them the spots on my skin. I then went to a dermatologist and turns out it was eczema. I was allergic to satin and had been wearing satin bras and panties and was breaking out. The disrespect and humiliation the doctor showed me by bringing people to look at me without asking, and their ignorance to not run any tests before making an assumption, the panic and stress they caused me thinking I had that disease, and their mindset to think the worst with me being an African American woman, was awful. The doctor was White. I don't remember if it was a man or a woman.

I had an accident—broke my wrist, which required immediate emergency surgery. My normal blood pressure stays at around 120/76, but my primary care doctor, the same doctor that tried to force me to get on a hypertension medication although I never had high blood pressure readings in her office, she DELAYED my surgery for twenty-four hours and FORCED me to see a cardiologist regarding "potential" hypertension due to my family history, and an article she read in a medical journal about hypertension in American Black families. Because of the unnecessary STRESS this doctor caused me—my blood pressure skyrocketed to 190/120. . . . I immediately threatened her with a lawsuit and fired her as my primary physician. The cardiologist tested me and gave the surgery center the okay for me to have surgery.

I was diagnosed with diverticulitis several years ago. The problem is it took three ER visits to finally get an answer. The first two doctors were White males. Though I was in severe pain, and I knew it wasn't normal, both told me I had a stomach bug and sent me home with meds. The final doctor was a Black male who was so compassionate, and said, I'm going to keep you here until we get to the bottom of this recurring issue. He ran extensive tests and kept me overnight. It was the best care I've ever experienced.

My father is a Black man. He started experiencing hypertension while he was relatively young. Given that he is a Black man, his doctors gave him a diagnosis of hypertension without any in-depth tests. For thirty years my father was active, ate healthy, but still had hypertension [and] took his meds. In 2010 he had a massive heart attack. He survived, but during his hospital stay he underwent routine blood work that found his potassium levels far below normal levels. This led to further investigations. He was found to have an extremely rare syndrome called Conn's syndrome, in which a tumor grows on the adrenal gland resulting in chronically low potassium levels [that] often lead to heart attacks and sometimes death. Though extremely rare, Conn's syndrome is easy to find through routine blood work. The type of blood work my dad had been undergoing for over thirty years. Had his primary doctor read through his blood work, they would have noticed his declining potassium levels over fifteen years ago.

I was actually dismissed by a doctor who is the same race that I am. I felt she felt too "common" with me and began to scold me like I was her aunt, or mother, and forgot about professionalism. It was her first time meeting me! I was thinking, you just met me.... You don't know me and shouldn't feel comfortable talking to me in that tone and manner.

I'm White. [My doctor] and his practice manager [his wife] are Black. His wife hates me and has charged me for services they didn't provide and threatened to cut me off if I didn't pay. The doctor doesn't like to be challenged by intelligent questions. He runs an assembly line practice and no longer takes the time to listen to me.

My former primary care doctor was an African American, as was her entire staff. Her staff made mistakes constantly with regard to insurance filings, appointments, forwarding messages to the doctor, etc. When I complained, the doctor took their side and accused me of complaining based on racial prejudice, even though I gave her specific examples of the office foul-ups. She actually "fired" me as a patient! That was a relief.

The Effect of Structural Racism

I believe that most health-care providers are *not* overtly or explicitly racists. In fact, most providers believe they treat all patients equally. Unfortunately, we live, work, and play in racist America. We live in a country where structural racism is endemic. No matter how much an individual health-care provider tries to ensure equal outcomes for all their patients, they cannot overcome the structural racism that surrounds them.

Structural racism generates and perpetuates inequities among races. It is woven into public policies, institutional practices, social forces, and ideologies. It runs deep in America, permeating education, law, finance, housing, and, of course, medicine. When a society allocates privilege on the basis of race, the health of individuals suffers.

I'll share an analogy to illustrate. I live in Maryland and love nature and gardening. Here, as throughout the country, we have a tree known as the Tree of Heaven (*Ailanthus altissima*.) As our state's most invasive tree, we call it the "Tree of Hell." Originally from China, it came to this country in 1784 and was valued back then as a sturdy street and shade tree. But the Tree of Heaven is rapidly spreading, and now has little value for lumber or wildlife nesting. It takes over an area, particularly one filled with sunshine, killing off other trees and shrubs. It does this by resprouting and root suckering as well as by producing a natural herbicide toxic to other species. Once cut or disturbed, the saplings send up hundreds of root suckers, often quite far from the parent tree. Some have been found growing up to two air miles from the nearest seed source. You have to kill the root to get rid of this tree.

You can see the parallel of the "Tree of Hell" with structural racism. Both are invasive, rapid-spreading, and toxic, but not indestructible. You just have to make sure to kill the root. Likewise, we have to kill the root causes of structural racism to eliminate medical racism. It's as simple and difficult as that.

A 2016 article in the *New England Journal of Medicine* shows how structural racism filters down to medical racism. The authors point out that measuring and assessing differences according to racial medical statistics, as is currently done by clinicians and health systems, can actually mask racism. It deflects attention away from underlying social causes, beyond biology, that may contribute to medical conditions. One example is diabetes, which has higher rates of complications among Black versus White Americans. "Successful treatment of such chronic conditions requires attention to structural factors and social determinants of health, but antiracism strategies are rarely recommended for improving diabetes control. Perhaps if we shift our clinical and research focus from race to racism, we can spur collective action rather than emphasizing only individual responsibility."

African Americans and Medical Racism

My experience is largely in how racism affects African Americans, since half of my practice is Black women. My own practice spurred me to take a deeper look into racism against Black Americans. Let's start with some facts:

- African Americans comprise 12.1 percent of the U.S. population.
- African American patients experience illness and infirmity at extremely high rates and have lower life expectancy than other racial and ethnic groups.
- Chronic illnesses associated with experiencing racism include heart attack, neurodegenerative disease, and metastatic cancer.
- African American patients are more likely to be uninsured than White Americans.
- African American patients spend almost double the percent of their family income on health-care premiums and out-of-pocket medical expenses than White Americans.

Nothing so starkly displays the force of medical racism as COVID. The CDC estimates Black individuals have died from COVID-19 at more than twice the rate of White individuals. Any old wives' tales about increased disease susceptibilities among non-White racial groups have been debunked. The evidence to date reaffirms that structural racism is a critical driving force behind COVID-19 disparities. In urban environments, studies suggest that fundamental causes of COVID-19 inequity include systemically racist policies and their inevitable downstream effects on housing, transportation, economic opportunity, education, food, air quality, health care, and beyond. Each of these social factors is associated with increased risk of COVID-19 exposure and increased case severity. From those social factors we get poor working conditions, limited access to health information or insurance, increased prevalence of comorbidities, cumulative life-course exposure to discrimination, low socioeconomic status, and other health risk conditions.

Seeing how health-care inequities flow from social inequities, we must know that we cannot treat our way out of public health crises even if treatment is equalized within our hospitals. Change will require comprehensive systems-level reforms and interventions. Clinicians, health systems, and policy makers alike must grapple with the fundamental inequities that lie upstream of disparate COVID-19 outcomes to make meaningful progress toward health justice.

Cardiovascular disease in African Americans is a primary cause of disparities in life expectancy between African Americans and Whites. African Americans have an earlier onset of cardiovascular disease, brought on by the higher prevalence of risk factors like hypertension, diabetes mellitus, obesity, and atherosclerotic heart disease. Hypertension is particularly prevalent and contributes directly to the increased risk of stroke, heart failure, and peripheral artery disease among African Americans. Disease management is less effective among African Americans, despite the availability of effective pharmacotherapies, including tailored pharmacotherapies for African Americans, such as heart failure medications. Ineffective disease management yields higher mortality. Explanations for these persistent disparities are multifactorial and span from the individual level to the social environment.

A study published in 2021 points out that for most cancers, Black people in the United States have both the highest death rate and shortest survival of any racial and ethnic group. The author notes, "Centuries of systemic deprivation of the Black population in the United States have yielded pervasive and long-lasting health consequences."

Multiple studies have shown that African American patients experience poorer surgical outcomes compared to White patients. The assumption is that preoperative surgical comorbidity, the simultaneous presence of two or more diseases or medical conditions in a patient, is the reason for this difference in adults. It is curious to note, however, that though healthy children historically have a low risk of postsurgical complications, research on more than 172,549 healthy children over a period of five years found that Black children had 3.43 times the odds of dying within thirty days after surgery and 18 percent greater odds of developing postoperative complications compared to White children. While the reasons for this are not clear, the researchers concluded that the difference could not be explained by racial differences in preoperative comorbidity.

Pain assessment is a central issue in medical racism against African Americans. As doctors, we know that assessment and treatment of pain is complicated. People experience pain differently and express it differently. In addition, assessment of pain is inherently subjective. When we can't attribute pain to an obvious source, such as traumatic injury, we providers have to rely on our own judgment, which can be influenced by our personal perceptions and biases. Providers are not immune to the media stereotypes that associate African Americans with substance abuse. In addition, in-group bias—identifying more with one's own group—also influences providers' ability to assess pain. A 2019 study that asked subjects to identify pain in facial photos found that White participants more readily recognized pain on White faces than on Black faces.

We can use clinical guidelines, standardized checklists, and system-wide protocols to leave less room for individual discretion—and therefore bias—to influence patient care. The Centers for Disease Control and Prevention (CDC) provides a *Guideline for Prescribing Opioids for Chronic Pain.* Released in 2016, it provides guidelines for when to initiate opioids for chronic pain, duration of use, dosage, and when to taper patients off opioids. To further avoid subjectivity in pain assessment, researchers are working to develop pain measures that move beyond a provider's interpretation of a patient's self-report, for example a blood test that can diagnose pain and its intensity using objective biomarkers. Although the research sounds intriguing, it seems to me the easier thing to do is to just believe the patient.

Remember my cousin Jarvis? He not only dressed up to see doctors, but he was also very careful about how he used language with them. "I am comfortable and confident in my ability to communicate with people no matter their level of expertise and education. Even when I don't know something, I can present as intelligent with some level of sophistication," he told me. "I do worry about people who don't have that ability to engage with the White world, the professional world and medical world."

So what are communication challenges for Black physicians? As a Black physician, especially one who grew up in poverty, it has been so enlightening to see how vastly communication styles differ between my community and most health-care providers. I have witnessed some of the most well-intentioned physicians, while trying to speak in laymen's terms, still miss the mark when communicating with Black and Brown patients. I contend that because of the lack of diversity in medical schools and training programs, there is a lack of diversity in health-care providers who can effectively communicate with patients who are not White.

Throughout my training, I was also keenly aware of medical mistrust that is prevalent in my community. In medical school, I was one of only four Black students to graduate in my class of over three hundred. I learned to modify aspects of my communication style to fit in better. I learned to "code switch," or alter my language, from the African American vernacular whenever I was in the presence of people who were not Black.

I had a patient, Ms. Jackson, who had been my patient for over a decade. She had a remote history of ovarian cancer but had been successfully treated for it years before. She had been going to get her yearly mammograms, but her gynecologist, who had followed her ovarian cancer, had been giving her the mammogram orders every year, so he was the one receiving the results. He was managing her breast health along with the cancer follow-up. One day, Ms. Jackson came to see me. She was someone who was very medically hesitant. She was resistant to taking any medication and mistrusted most medical professionals, even me at times. During our entire visit, she seemed a little anxious. Finally, at the end of the visit, I asked, "Is everything okay? Is there something else you'd like to talk about?"

She began to tell me, "I had something wrong with my mammogram, so they did a biopsy. Now the doctor keeps calling my phone saying I have cancer and need chemotherapy!" I immediately thought, how inappropriate of them to call and give this patient cancer results over the phone? Why didn't they contact me, her primary care doctor of over ten years? I knew Ms. Jackson had a tremendous amount of medical hesitancy, but I had developed a rapport with her. It turns out that they did call and give her the cancer diagnosis over the phone. It was only after she refused to come in to speak with the doctor that they mentioned what treatment she might need to take, including the possibility of chemotherapy.

I started talking to Ms. Jackson in my "doctor voice" but soon realized that I was not using the expressions and colloquialisms that would make her comfortable. I code-switched back into my original African American communication style. "I understand that you're not trying to claim breast cancer." "Exactly!" she responded. I realized that Ms. Jackson felt that if she didn't "claim" the cancer, it wouldn't be so. This is a popular denial tactic that we sometimes experience in the Black community. I see it often with diabetes, where patients often insist, "I'm not claiming diabetes." Ms. Jackson wanted to pretend that the cancer did not exist. What she really needed was for someone to speak to her in person, and it needed to be someone she felt comfortable with and trusted. After I explained everything to her, she expressed understanding and acceptance and agreed to seek treatment for the newly diagnosed, early-stage cancer. I am happy to say that she is alive and well three years later.

Medical Racism and Other Groups

Medical racism can take the form of microaggressions, intentional or unintentional verbal, behavioral, or environmental slights that communicate hostile, derogatory, or negative attitudes toward a stigmatized or culturally marginalized group. Patients are left feeling disrespected, distrustful, and hesitant to participate in shared decision-making with their doctors.

While I knew about microaggressions toward African Americans, Native Americans, and Hispanics, I was surprised to find out that Asian American patients also felt them and were more likely than White American patients to report that their health-care providers did not treat them with respect. Asian Americans are perceived as immigrants even though many have lived in the United States for generations. "Asian Americans report being told that they speak English well (the assumption being that English could not possibly be their first language) and being asked where they are from (with the questioner often responding incredulously when an Asian American says they are from a particular US city or state)." The researchers reported that some Asian Americans felt victimized by the "all Asians look alike" assumption, which ignores Asian subgroups such as Chinese, Japanese, or Korean, important differences that should be understood by health-care providers.

Like Asian Americans, the Hispanic and Latinx populations represent many different countries and cultures. The largest ethnic minority in the United States, they have the highest numbers of uninsured of any group, although their life expectancies exceed non-Hispanic Whites. Medical bias against Hispanic and Latinx patients occurs not only because of poverty and assumptions about their immigration status but also through a lack of understanding of cultural differences. For example, nursing and medical students described Hispanic patients as less compliant than White or Asian patients and perceived them as having more family involvement in health care.

Physicians cited difficulty in communicating health-related information to Hispanic and Latinx patients as a barrier to care. Some health-care professionals also associated the group with risky health behaviors such as unsafe sexual practices or smoking. The researchers felt that the health-care workers' training in "cultural competency" may have instilled these stereotypes, increasing rather than reducing bias.

I was moved by a presentation by Dr. Kimberly Manning, an internist at Grady Hospital in Atlanta, Georgia. Dr. Manning, who is also a diversity, equity, and inclusion expert, shared a patient story that was a great example of approaching a different culture in a creative way. A woman was hospitalized for a severe illness and was going to miss a milestone birthday celebration. Dr. Manning brought in a balloon to lift her spirits, but the patient was still sad and upset. Then the doctor pulled out her cell phone and played "Las Mañanitas," a song that a Mexican colleague had played for her birthday. The patient could not stop laughing and smiling. A Black doctor had truly acknowledged her with a gesture that meant so much in her culture. Dr. Manning, who is African American, has also realized that diversity, equity, and inclusion is for everyone—not just for Black people.

Native Americans have also experienced medical racism. The severely underfunded Indian Health Service (IHS) is meant to provide care to over 2.2 million Native Americans from more than 560 recognized tribes, a legal obligation of the United States in fulfillment of treaty promises. IHS's long-term inadequacies have resulted in tribal members' poor health conditions. According to an analysis by the National Congress of American Indians, if the IHS were to match the level of care provided to federal prisoners, government funding would have to be nearly doubled. Even higher funding would be required for IHS to match the benefits guaranteed to other Americans by programs like Medicaid.

Native Americans also face a shortage of health-care providers. This problem exists in many rural American communities, but it is particularly severe in remote reservation locations. Doctors often do not see Native American patients until they are much sicker than their White counterparts. Native Americans and Alaska Natives have a life expectancy of 6.5 years less than the United States' other races combined. They continue to die at higher rates from preventable diseases like chronic liver disease and cirrhosis, diabetes, and chronic lower respiratory diseases.

I see similarities between African Americans and Native Americans. In addition to shared poverty levels, lack of adequate food and housing, and other social determinants of health, both groups have suffered extreme trauma, prejudice, and persecution by White America. In 2021, the National Diversity Council hosted its first Native American Summit, featuring a panel on historical deficiencies in health care among Native American and Alaskan Natives. I was struck by how similar the history of trauma during sanctioned government actions against Native Americans was, to what occurred to African Americans, and the effect it has had on their health.

A U.S. government–published fact sheet, "Understanding Historical Trauma When Responding to an Event in Indian Country," was written for disaster behavioral health responders to understand the effect of historical trauma on disaster preparedness and response efforts for Native Americans. To quote the document: "The effects of historical trauma among Native Americans include changes in the traditional ways of child rearing, family structure, and relationships. Some observed responses to historical trauma may include signs of overall poor physical health and depression, substance abuse, and high rates of suicide. In many cases, historical trauma has also disrupted the sense of community within the tribe itself. There is a well-founded mistrust of outsiders and government providers based on long-term negative experiences with non–Native Americans."

While acknowledging historical trauma, this document also perpetuates stereotypes and medical racism. It fails to acknowledge the kinship and extended family relationships that are at the core of Native American cultures. It fails to acknowledge the belief that each generation is responsible to teach the next generation values, tradition, and beliefs and keep tribal languages, ceremonies, and customs alive. It fails to share the spiritual aspects of Native American culture and deep ties to nature that are part of both mental and physical health. While the intention is to build the providers' cultural competency, it actually encourages racism.

Medical Racism and Religion

While religions are not generally seen as a race or ethnicity, both patients and health-care providers can experience medical racism based on their religion. Numerous studies have shown the strong bias in health care against Muslim doctors and patients in America. Members of other religious sects often feel that their beliefs are not honored by health-care practitioners. For example, preventative practices such as vaccination may have lower vaccination rates by followers of specific religions, even though very few religions actually prohibit use of vaccinations. This puts religious beliefs in direct conflict with public health.

In almost all cases, doctors are required to override religious beliefs if a patient requires an emergency procedure and refuses medical care. For example, Jehovah's Witnesses consider blood transfusions to be against God's will. Legally, doctors cannot force them to have this procedure if it is not an emergency. But if it is an emergency, or if the individual is in a severely altered mental state, then medicine takes precedent over religion. This issue becomes particularly controversial in the case of children. While an adult can refuse care for themselves, refusing care for their children often ends up in the courts. Members of the Followers of Christ, for instance, refuse all medical care in favor of faith-healing. They will not go to a hospital even if it is a matter of life or death. But when they bring that belief system into parenting, generally authorities step in.

So the question is: Should we call this medical racism when an individual's decision-making rights are taken away because the government intervenes based on what is perceived as more worthy moral and ethical values? Historically, religion and health care have been highly interconnected. It is just in the last few centuries that there has been a clearer separation between medicine and religion with medicine being aligned with evidence-based research and religion holding the reins on spiritual and moral health. One of the biggest areas of government intervention is in the area of reproductive rights, where religious influences and government laws become highly intertwined.

For most patients, religious beliefs and medicine clash at a time when they are most vulnerable. Health-care providers can unwittingly approach diagnosis and treatment in a way that goes against an individual's religious commitment. This often occurs when patients are turning to their religious and spiritual beliefs in making medical decisions. I believe strongly that it is important for health-care providers to apply the same compassion, empathy, and respect to religious and spiritual needs as well. This requires cultural competency training to understand those beliefs, so knowledge can improve patient-provider communications.

This knowledge can fall into areas such as prayer, diet, medicines, and more. For example, many religions believe that prayer assists in healing. Are we providing an environment and uninterrupted time that allows for prayer? Some religions have dietary restrictions on eating or using medicines that contain pork products. Are we providing alternatives that enhance healing? Other religions have rituals relating to end-of-life or use of certain drugs during that time. How are we handling different beliefs during this extremely vulnerable time? Still others have strong rules about women and men interacting. Are we providing same-gender health-care practitioners whenever possible?

Understanding the tenets of religion and their clinical significance is complicated but important. As the authors of *Cultural Religious Competence in Clinical Practice* explain: "Listening to a patient's beliefs along with how those beliefs are tied to the patient's health can help build a positive relationship between the health practitioner and patient. Knowledge of religious and spiritual beliefs and practices can result in decreased medical errors, earlier patient release, and reliable communication between patient and health-care provider that results in improved health-care delivery."

Cultural Competency versus Cultural Humility

Cultural competency and antibias training are now required for many, but not all, health-care providers. Cultural competency training assumes that the more knowledge we have about another race or ethnicity, the more competent we will be in practice. But as we saw with the government fact sheet on Native Americans, some "cultural competency" training perpetuates stereotyping and bias. An alternative movement works toward training in cultural humility and sensitivity, which assumes that we can never teach people everything they need to know about another culture. Health-care providers can never become fully culturally competent at a group level, so humility training aims to teach health-care providers that every individual patient is different and changing, not an amalgam of cultural stereotypes. We need to acknowledge our own bias as providers. We can't get rid of our bias entirely, but we can humbly acknowledge it and remove it as much as possible from our patients' experience.

What do we need to do to mitigate medical racism based on the idea of cultural humility? I think it comes down to three core strategies. First, we need to be aware of health-related beliefs, practices, and cultural values in diverse populations. Our patients might bring their cultures' traditional practices and treatments with them to our examining table. We are challenged to acknowledge those cultural practices while still basing our approach on evidence-based research and sensitivity to the individual, but that respect is necessary if we are to build trust between providers and patients. Second, we must look at the diagnostic and treatment data for each population and subpopulation. We can't treat all Asian Americans, for example, the same. Finally, we need to LISTEN more, with genuine curiosity to our patients as individuals, acknowledging our own biases and their histories. Then we can work toward building a no-judgment zone in our practices. Our no-judgment zone needs to go beyond race and ethnicity. Bias relating to gender identity and sexual orientation also results in inequitable health care. And when race and gender meet as the target for bias, the consequences to the lives of individuals are significant.

CHAPTER 8

Dismissing Women, Gender Identity, and Sexual Orientation

W HEN I STARTED MY PRIMARY medicine practice devoted to women's health twenty years ago, nobody else was doing that. Even today, few such practices exist in the United States. We tend to think women's health is just about obstetrics and gynecology, but cis women are not men with female parts. We are anatomically, physiologically, mentally, and emotionally different than men through and through. Every cell in our bodies expresses women's genes. Yet when it comes to women's health, the medical field focuses on the things that make us different from men—our breasts and vaginas. And as women, we do too. We'll get our pap smears and mammograms done before we have our heart tested or cholesterol checked, even though heart disease is the number one killer of women—not breast or cervical cancer.

It's called "bikini medicine," which is medical practice, research, and funding focused solely on the female breasts and reproductive system. I'm not fond of the term, since I'm not fond of bikinis, but it does tell it like it is. The implicit bias of bikini medicine has led to inadequacies in the diagnosis and treatment of major diseases that affect women—heart disease, cancer, and diabetes. It has led to dismissal of majority-female autoimmune diseases like lupus, which for many years was considered a condition "all in HER mind." Auto-immune diseases are now a silent epidemic in America, with one in six people coping with the range of conditions, 75 percent of whom are women. Bikini medicine's anatomical hyperfocus also ignores depression and anxiety, which women are twice as likely to suffer, along with its ripple effects on their physical health.

Working with Women

From early in my career, I have felt that women need special attention from health care. We present with different symptoms in some diseases than men. ("Present" means to show the symptoms a doctor looks for in a particular condition.) Women are dismissed and ultimately have worse outcomes because the medical community is looking for "man symptoms," whereas we have "woman symptoms." Many of our symptoms are less specific and more diffuse, indicative of a number of different possible underlying conditions. Women require deeper investigation from their doctors.

I have learned that listening to and believing my patients is vital. The number one complaint I hear from new patients is that their past doctors did not listen. Equally important, I work to make my women patients understand that it is *their responsibility* to listen to and believe in their bodies. I often see patients who say, "It's been bothering me for months, but I didn't think it was a big deal." We women tend to devalue our feelings, both emotional and physical. Your body knows and tells you things. Pay attention. I have met many more women who underestimated their symptoms than overestimated. We need to be realists and truth-seekers. For many women, their emotional state dictates how they feel about their health. For example, a person with a cheerful mood thinks their health is better than it is, where a depressed person may feel that they are sicker than they really are. To start getting healthy, we need to find the truth. That goes back to learning about our bodies, listening to them, and working closely with our health-care team.

I believe women are more proactive about their health than men. They seem to listen more, be more compliant, and are truly concerned about health-care matters. I still remember a dialogue with a guy patient (I occasionally take a male patient who is related to one of my female patients) who asked me, "Why didn't you open up a men's practice?" I responded jokingly, "Because it would be empty. Men don't see doctors." I know that's not entirely true, but I choose to do women's health because I've found that women care about their health and follow recommendations.

My women patients are often caregivers for their families and other people in their communities. They are more vulnerable because of all the things they do for others, sometimes at the expense of their own health. They are often working more hours for less pay on top of their unpaid caregiver roles. Research shows that caregivers take less care of their own health than that of the people they care for. They dismiss their own needs. My unique medical practice, Comprehensive Women's Health, is designed to give women the special care they need as women and as caregivers.

Hypertension, heart disease, and diabetes are the three physical conditions I see most in my patients. I also see more anxiety and depression than other primary care practices. I am not surprised to see these physical and mental health conditions arise so frequently in my women patients. I know these problems are rooted in the challenges of lifestyle and socioeconomic factors that affect women more than men.

Women have clear selection criteria when they choose a doctor. In our Pulse Survey, 86 percent of respondents said how the doctor listened to them was important to their physician choice, followed by 79 percent on how the doctor explained things, and 69 percent on the doctor's reputation and knowledge. Interestingly, only 29 percent cared how friendly the medical professional was, and 25 percent factored in a recommendation from a family member or friend. Sixty-nine percent considered shared gender more important than shared race or ethnicity in selecting a doctor.

I was not surprised that 50 percent of women respondents believed that their gender was a reason they had been treated differently by a medical professional. Actual survey comments provided additional perspectives on gender biases:

Previous doctors were male. Females listen better to females.

My worst experience has been with male doctors, who do not listen, walk into the room, criticize without understanding, [and] leave me feeling helpless and frustrated.

When I was worried [that] a lump [I found] might be breast cancer and my aunt just passed from breast cancer, and the male doctor was grinning like he wanted to laugh.

As a teenager, I had a period of time where I suffered debilitating headaches almost daily and also heavy and painful periods. I did not have a GYN then, just a regular doctor. He basically called me a moody teenager. In fact, I suffered from severe allergies that when treated, helped with the migraine and PCOS.

I was losing two units of blood/period, so anemic that I was being evaluated for blood cancer, and two gynecologists, one primary care physician, and a hematologist (all male) couldn't connect the two because they thought I was exaggerating my monthly blood loss. (The issue was a submucosal fibroid, well known for creating massive blood loss.)

Had a gynecologist call me sweety during an appointment and consult, where he performed a gyn exam and discussed cancer treatment and possible surgery. Never once used my name.

Male oncologist would not listen to my side effects. Would never answer my questions about care or my questions about my care plan.

The Slowly Changing World of Women's Health

Things have improved somewhat over the last few decades for the overall health of women. More money is being spent on research, and there is more inclusion of women in clinical trials. More attention is being paid to mental health. At least 50 percent of medical students are now women. There is more focus on health issues for women of different races and ethnicities, as well as how social determinants affect women's health. Women are finding their voices, becoming increasingly vocal about their diagnosis and treatment—witness the #MeToo movement.

While overt sexism in the United States has diminished, bias against women is still prevalent. Policies are still driven by the White men who hold power in academia, research, business, and government. Their religious or political agendas can be ignorant of and harmful to the health of women, as in the continuing assault on female reproductive rights.

Social determinants of health also continue to play a disproportionate role in women's health. Most people living in poverty in the United States are women, and we know the profound effect of poverty on health outcomes. I am very concerned about the racial and ethnic disparities in maternal morbidity and mortality. Black women are three to four times more likely to die from pregnancy-related disease than white women. This is not a new issue in the United States, but the gap between Whites and non-Whites in severe maternal morbidities and mortality has widened over the last few decades. Non-Hispanic Black women had the fastest rate of increase in maternal deaths between 2007 and 2014, with maternal death rates up to twelve times higher in some cities than Non-Hispanic White women. Pregnancy-related mortality is also higher among Native Americans/ Native Alaskans, Asians/Pacific Islanders, and for certain subgroups of Hispanic women, such as Puerto Ricans in some regions of the United States.

For example, researchers believe that structural racism plays a large role in these disparities and recommend a comprehensive approach to the reproductive care of women, from preconception through the periods between pregnancies. "Comprehensive" means women's health does not begin with pregnancy and end with the birth of a child. A comprehensive approach would consider all our parts throughout our lifespans. It would include emotional, intellectual, and spiritual well-being along with physical health. This sort of approach is best suited to primary care.

Unfortunately, problems with our primary health-care system prevent the advance of a comprehensive model. A 2020 report by the Commonwealth Fund, a private foundation whose mission is to promote a high-performing health-care system, found that gaps and barriers in the primary health-care system inhibit meeting the needs of women across their lives. Among those were medical training, biases, time constraints, lack of focus on social factors, competing professional and personal obligations, language, culture, lack of a regular source of primary care, underrepresentation of women in health-care leadership and policymaking, and the politicization of women's health issues. The report outlined three areas where primary health-care systems can better serve women at all stages of life: care relating to health needs unique to women, like pregnancy and menopause; gender-tailored diagnosis and treatment of women for conditions like heart disease and neurodegenerative diseases; and care specific to lesbian, gay, bisexual, transgender, queer, intersex, and asexual (LGBTQIA) health needs.

A Major Setback to Women's Health

As I was writing this book, the U.S. Supreme Court overturned *Roe v. Wade*. This is a major setback for women's health. While there are states that allow abortion, we now do not have a national policy and protection on an issue that the majority of Americans support—a woman's right to choose. Most women count on the freedom to choose when to bear children and do not want the government to intervene with this right. Quite simply, we have experienced a major denial to our personal freedoms relating to procreation. This is beyond alarming. It is horrifying.

I have seen many patients who are literally sick over this decision. They are depressed and anxious. I've even had some women who are so disturbed by this ruling that they are contemplating moving to another country. At least sixty-five countries have legalized or decriminalized abortion on request, including our neighbors, Mexico and Canada. Are my patients' reactions overly dramatic? I don't think so. This decision cancels our rights and dismisses our concerns, which is appalling for a country that claims to hold individual freedoms in such high regard.

Beyond the emotional and mental toll of having choice taken away, women are now faced with very real physical and financial consequences. Those consequences also affect the men in their lives, their families, and their communities. Have we forgotten the thousands of pregnancy-related deaths from illegal abortions? Do we really believe that economic potential and career opportunities for women will not be affected by taking away their right to choose? Can we ignore a decision that will cause the most harm to Black, Latinx, Indigenous, and other people of color who already experience systemic racism and lack of access to health care? Will we continue to ignore the historical fact that restricted abortion access does not change the number of unintended pregnancies or reduce demand for abortion?

My hope is that by the time you are reading this book, legislation will give back what should never have been taken away. We must change this ultimate dismissal of women.

Medical Bias and LGBTQIA People

With increasing awareness of gender identity and sexual orientation, health care has an increased need for self-education aimed toward unbiased treatment. These issues were not even talked about when I was in medical school. Historically, America (and most of the world) has ignored the fact that not all humans identify simply as men or women. Our historically rigid definitions of gender and sexuality affect the health of millions of Americans. An estimated 5.6 percent of Americans identify as lesbian, gay, bisexual, transgender, or queer, with nearly 16 percent of Generation Z (18 to 23) considering themselves something other than cis heterosexual. That number compares to just 2 percent of Americans fifty-six and older. Out of 330 million adult Americans, a lot of people are being dismissed.

Many medical professionals are struggling to understand the fluid nature of gender identity and sexual orientation. We may find ourselves googling terms such as "cisgender," "genderqueer," "intersex," "pansexual" or "non-binary." Some of us bristle at the need to reshape our language to use "they" instead of "he" or "she." Others work hard to be aware of gender identity and chose words carefully. We are grateful when our patients correct us.

Not just the medical community but society as a whole must face its biases about sexuality and gender identity. In American mainstream culture we don't talk openly about sex and gender. Human sexuality has always been a spectrum rather than just a duality. We cannot deny the rights of any human individuals simply because we see them as "other." By denying the existence of the many points on the spectrum of gender identification and sexual orientation, mainstream society has caused them pain and suffering. We in medicine are among the guilty.

Treating Lesbian and Bisexual Women

When I started my practice, most of my patients were heterosexual women. Later, when I began treating lesbians and bisexual women, both as individuals and couples, I learned that many had been dismissed by other medical professionals, not always with explicit bias but often with implicit bias. Their sexuality as lesbians or bisexual women was ignored. As their primary doctor, I resolved to acknowledge all my patients' concerns, including their gender and sexuality. Today I have a number of lesbian patients who are more comfortable with me than they were with other doctors. With me they know that no part of their lives will be dismissed. They speak freely about their relationships and their ongoing struggle to claim their right to a place in "normal" society.

Research has shown increased health risks for lesbian and bisexual women. They have a greater risk of breast and gynecologic cancers because they are less likely to have regular cancer screenings and have higher rates of obesity, both of which are linked to cancer. They are more likely to smoke, use drugs, or drink—all of which are linked to cancer, lung disease, and heart disease, the three top causes of death among women. The health and behavior gaps between lesbian and heterosexual women appear to be narrowing, but so far there are few longitudinal studies tracking these advances. One study in Pittsburgh, Pennsylvania, followed more than one thousand women over ten years. The baseline survey reported higher rates of obesity, depression, and smoking among lesbian participants than heterosexual women, but ten years later only smoking remained as a higher risk factor. We need further research like this to help us better serve our patients of all orientations.

Treating Patients Who Identify as Transgender

I have no transgender women in my practice currently, so my understanding of their issues comes from research and anecdotes from other medical professionals. From those sources I have learned that bias against transgender people in the United States is prevalent and is the cause of health disparities.

Transgender individuals face social stigma, discrimination from the world around them, as well as their own internalization of negative social attitudes. Transgender people tend to receive less preventive care than cisgender people. This could be from fear of discrimination, gender-based insurance coverage, being refused care, or difficulty finding a doctor with expertise in transgender care. They are also more at risk of emotional and psychological abuse, physical and sexual violence, hepatitis and HIV, substance misuse, and mental health problems.

In 2010, a landmark survey by the National Center for Transgender Equality quantified the high levels of poverty, discrimination, and violence faced by transgender people. Five years later, a follow-up survey of twenty-eight thousand transgender adults again presented a troubling picture:

- Individuals who identify as transgender live in poverty at more than twice the rate of the general population. For transgender people of color, the poverty rate is three times the "normal" rate.
- Thirty percent of respondents reported being fired, denied a promotion, or being otherwise mistreated on the job because of their gender identity.

- One third had experienced homelessness.
- One quarter had experienced housing discrimination.
- One third reported at least one negative experience with a health-care provider, such as verbal harassment or refusal of treatment because of their gender identity.

Implicit bias can emerge in our interaction with transgender people, even for those of us who are conscious of our bias issues and working to keep them separate from our behavior. I recently viewed a medical lecture given by Dr. Kimberly Manning, a diversity and inclusion expert. Dr. Manning tells of a patient visit at a primary care clinic, part of a "safety net" hospital that did not require insurance. A new patient had just arrived in the area and needed to establish a primary care doctor to get her medications refilled. Seeing that the prescriptions were for gender-affirming hormones, Dr. Manning told the new patient that she didn't feel qualified to refill them herself but could refer the patient to endocrinologists. Those providers would require health insurance, unlike the clinic.

The new patient challenged her: "Do you tell your patients with hyperthyroidism that you don't know enough about it? Is that what you do when you encounter something new? What would you do with a patient who did not have insurance?" The patient got up to leave, having faced such discouraging treatment before. Dr. Manning then realized that by referring away this patient she would be abandoning her goal of patient-focused care. Her definition of primary care had been too narrow. She made the calls she needed to educate herself on how to care for this patient. From then on, she would include transgender patients with all the other unique individuals in her care. This is a model we should all strive toward—being able to recognize our bias and self-correct for the benefit of our patients. I greatly appreciate Dr. Manning for allowing herself to be vulnerable enough to share that compelling story. I have also since undergone cultural bias training around transgender patients in order to better understand their life lens so that I will be prepared for my future patients.

Health and Discrimination for Gay and Bisexual Men

I was a young teenager when AIDS began its devastation. I was unaware of the homophobia ingrained in our culture. I knew nothing of the Stonewall Riots of 1969, which ignited the Gay Rights Movement and established that gay men would no longer tolerate being invisible and shamed in America. I was too busy coping with what it meant to be Black and living in poverty in this country. Since then, I have seen the AIDS epidemic's dual effects of raising awareness of LGBTQIA issues and revealing antigay bias.

Nearly 330,000 gay and bisexual men with stage 3 HIV (AIDS) have died in the United States since the 1980s, when it was considered an acute fatal disease with a life expectancy of just weeks or months. Fortunately, things have changed dramatically. Today HIV/AIDS is a manageable chronic disease: A twenty-year-old with HIV can expect to live to seventy. Medicine has made great strides in antiretroviral therapies, but HIV/AIDS prevention and access to treatment are still issues, particularly in younger gay and bisexual African American and Latino men. More than half of the people with HIV are gay or bisexual men, and most new cases are occurring in this group.

The stress of discrimination increases the likelihood of physical and mental disorders in gay and bisexual men. Research has shown that they are more likely to abuse tobacco and alcohol, increasing risk of cancers and liver damage. They have higher rates of sexually transmitted infections such as HPV and gonorrhea. Gay and bisexual men also have increased incidence of major depression, bipolar disorder, and generalized anxiety disorder, particularly if they are struggling to hide their sexuality. In supportive settings, it helps to be "out"—men who are open about their sexual orientation have better health outcomes than closeted gay and bisexual men. Hiding and fear of disclosure add to stress. In less supportive settings, however, being "out" can invite discrimination along with its damage to mental health.

The CDC Speaks Out on LGBT

The CDC's social health data analysis confirms that individuals who identify as LGBT (this is the term used by CDC) face health disparities from societal stigma, discrimination, and denial of their civil and human rights, which can in turn result in psychiatric disorders, substance abuse, and suicide. It confirms that violence and victimization have long-term effects on individuals who identify as LGBT and our society. They acknowledge that personal, family, and social acceptance of sexual orientation and gender identity can affect the mental health and personal safety of individuals who identify as LGBT.

The CDC recommends these actions to improve LGBT health:

• Increased collection of sexual orientation and gender identity (SOGI) data on health surveys and records.
• Promoting open and supportive patient-provider interaction. Providers should inquire about and be supportive of sexual orientation and gender identity.
• Providing medical students with better training in LGBT issues.
• Implementing anti-bullying policies in schools.
• Providing services to reduce suicide and homelessness among youth. (LGBT youth are two to three times more likely to attempt suicide and more likely to experience homelessness.)
• Improved interventions to curb HIV and other sexually transmitted infections.

Becoming Leaders to Instigate Change

I am fortunate to have had others who paved the way for me to be-come a Black woman physician and then pay it forward. As the great Maya Angelou said: "I've learned that you shouldn't go through life with a catcher's mitt on both hands. You need to be able to throw something back." Helping individuals overcome barriers, however, is just a part of the societal change required to ensure the rights of people who have been historically dismissed—including the right to equitable health care. This broader societal change cannot occur until members of the dismissed groups hold decision-making and leader-ship positions. Allies can help, but it takes leaders who have walked in the shoes of the oppressed to break down systemic barriers.

Even though women make up 80 percent of the health-care work-force, they are woefully underrepresented in leadership positions. Less than 20 percent of hospital leadership roles are held by women. Only 4 percent of health-care companies have a female CEO. In the companies considered most influential in health care, only 21 percent of board members are women. Women make up only 18 percent of department chairs in academic medicine. Only 27 percent of Con-gress is made up of women. The percentage of individuals who identify as LGBTQIA in leadership positions is miniscule.

The picture for women doctors is a bit better. More than 53.7 per-cent of the students matriculating into medical schools are now women. That is a good thing for patients: Female physicians tend to provide more preventive care, score higher on empathy scales, and follow clinical guidelines more often than their male counterparts, resulting in better patient outcomes, fewer hospital readmissions, and lower mortality rates. These new women physicians will provide new leadership in the medical profession, influencing research and education as well as patient care.

Yet, many specialties still lack women, and that may affect patient outcomes. One study discovered that if their surgeon is male, women are 32 percent more likely to die, 20 percent more likely to stay in the hospital longer, and 16 percent more likely to have complications. The study, which analyzed data from more than 1.3 million Canadian patients who underwent twenty-one different kinds of common elective surgeries, concluded that there is a need for more women surgeons because they may get better outcomes by working with women patients differently, talking with them more after surgery, and consulting with other specialists. The challenge, they concluded, is the culture of medicine and surgery makes it harder for women to become surgeons.

Additionally, we must keep women doctors in practice after they graduate. Female physicians experience 60 percent more burnout than male physicians. Existing challenges to work-life balance have been aggravated by the demands of the COVID pandemic, but one study suggests that burnout also results because female doctors have more female patients than male doctors, and more patients with psychosocial complexity. They suggest that the burnout problem among female physicians could be reduced by increasing visit time, training in patient expectations during medical school, adjusting for patient gender in compensation and reimbursement plans, and including behavioral medicine specialists on primary care teams. These measures would also work toward improving health-care outcomes for women and the LGBTQIA community.

Bias against women and the LGBTQIA population has existed throughout history. Mainstream awareness of it may be new, but for those who have experienced mistreatment, it is all too familiar. Sometimes, I feel that change moves at a glacial pace, and we take two steps back for every one step forward. But I have seen enough positive momentum in my years practicing medicine to know that while the mountain is steep, we can still reach the top.

CHAPTER 9

The Perils of Ageism

M Y AUNT JANE IS NINETY-FIVE years old. She served as a Lt. Colonel in the United States Air Force and was one of the first three African American women to complete the United States Air Force Officer Candidate School. After retiring from the military, she earned a doctorate from George Washington University, had a second career at the American Red Cross, was the first Black area vice president of AARP, traveled to all seven continents, and wrote her autobiography when she was ninety-two. She is a formidable and accomplished woman.

Chances are that Jane would be invisible to many Americans. Many would see her as just another older Black woman. That's what happens in our society when you get old. We forget that senior people have lived rich and often extraordinary lives. We act like they landed on this planet as old people and fail to show them respect. Ageism is real. It lies beneath the dismissal and neglect of older people in our youth-obsessed country. When older people are dismissed or short-changed in health care, they suffer unnecessary physical, emotional, and mental consequences.

We tend to rank biases based on our own experiences. Of course we're appalled by racism. Most of us have spoken out against discrimination against women. But the bias of ageism, like aging people, gets dismissed as less important by those of us who have yet to get old. It is so ubiquitous that it seems normal. In fact, 82 percent of older Americans report experiencing ageism regularly. Sixty-five percent have experienced ageist messages from the media. Forty-five percent report having experienced interpersonal ageism, and 36 percent report having internalized ageism, believing it themselves.

I'm lucky to have many senior patients, and this is what I believe: There's nothing different between them and me other than they've been here longer. If I'm lucky, I'll get there someday too. I try to give them grace, respect, and a little bit of extra attention. I try to do my part to alleviate the pain of the misconceptions and dismissal they face as they age.

Misconceptions about Aging

One misconception about seniors is that they are all unhealthy. Actually, more than 40 percent of people over sixty-five report that they are in good or excellent health. That's a good thing, since the average life expectancy of Americans is almost eighty years.

Another misconception is that people are living longer primarily because of medical intervention. While there is some basis for this belief (a hundred years ago, the average life expectancy was fifty-nine, so medicine does keep people alive), there are many other factors that keep people living good lives longer. One of my favorite studies on aging is the Blue Zone Project, which has been going on since 2008. The project is working to discover the lifestyles that lead to vitality and longevity. An interdisciplinary team of researchers looked at the five areas in the world with the highest percentage of centenarians. These areas, which were dubbed the Blue Zones, are in Loma Linda, California, USA; Nicoya, Costa Rica; Sardinia, Italy; Ikaria, Greece; and Okinawa, Japan. What began as a National Geographic expedition, lead by Dan Buettner, to uncover the secrets of longevity and evolved into the discovery of the five places around the world where people consistently live over 100 years, dubbed the Blue Zones. Dan and his team of demographers, scientist, and anthropologists were able to distill the evidence-based common denominators of these Blue Zones into nine commonalities that they call the Power 9. They have since taken these principles into communities across the United States, working with policy makers, local businesses, schools, and individuals to shape the environments of the Blue Zones Project Communities. What has been found is that putting the responsibility of curating a healthy environment on an individual does not work, but through policy and environmental changes, the Blue Zones Project Communities have been able to increase life expectancy, reduce obesity, and make the healthy choice the easy choice for millions of Americans.

The researchers have identified nine lifestyle characteristics that help these people live longer and better. One group of recommendations is no surprise: Be physically active, stop eating before you are full, eat a primarily plant-based diet, and drink alcohol moderately. Other longevity factors are more surprising: Seniors need to have a purpose. Knowing your purpose is worth up to seven years of extra life expectancy. Further, the longest-lived people in the world have routines to handle stress. Stress is inevitable and leads to the chronic inflammation associated with every major age-related disease. But these long-lived seniors know how to handle it. It is also important to belong to a faith-based community and a social circle that supports healthy behaviors. And people in the Blue Zones put their families first, have lifelong partners, and live with or near children and grandchildren.

Connection, purpose, and support are foundational to people who are aging well. The medical community often fails to recognize these social factors, focusing on medical diagnosis and treatment rather than on a holistic physical, emotional, spiritual, and mental approach to health.

A third misconception about aging is that you inevitably become less "sharp." While aging does affect cognitive functions, most people over sixty-five do not lose their thinking ability. According to the CDC, cognitive decline among adults aged sixty-five years and older is 11.7 percent, compared to 10.8 percent among adults 45–64 years of age. When health-care providers assume senior patients are mentally impaired, they can make poor judgment calls. That's what happened to Sarah, a friend of my aunt Jane.

Sarah was in her late eighties, a very intelligent, clear-headed woman who held a master's degree and had enjoyed a successful career. She was hospitalized with very severe circulation problems in her legs that had caused an infection. The blood flow to her legs was so bad that her doctors said they would need to be amputated, assuming that Sarah would be mentally incapable of participating in alternative treatment decisions. Sarah was sent home with a prognosis of losing her legs.

Sarah reached out and told me that the doctors in the hospital had talked down to her as if she were unintelligent, or as a child. She felt strongly that they had not done a thorough job looking at other options. After reviewing her medical records, I introduced her to a different vascular surgeon. He did additional testing and was able save her legs. Sarah passed away a few years later, but I am so grateful that she did not have to live her remaining life with an unnecessary amputation.

What Is Ageism?

Our population is rapidly aging. It is estimated that between 2015 and 2050 the proportion of the world's older adults will almost double from 12 percent to 22 percent. This means two billion people will be over the age of sixty and living longer lives. This is a major issue both for individuals and for society.

I can see three intertwined manifestations of ageism. *Institutional* ageism occurs when an institution perpetuates ageism through its practices and policies. Second, *interpersonal* ageism is shown in biases in personal and professional interactions. Third, with *internalized* ageism, a person internalizes ageist beliefs and applies them to themselves. Since one's attitudes about age may influence their health behaviors, ageist beliefs could lead to a fatalism about inevitable decay and so a neglect of self-care.

All three types of ageism play out in health-care systems and interactions. Multiple studies show that ageism leads to adverse outcomes and increased mortality. For example, in a study of nine thousand hospitalized patients, researchers found that health-care professionals were more likely to withhold life-sustaining treatments from older patients compared with younger ones, even after controlling for prognosis and patient preferences.

Like other forms of discrimination, ageism manifests in explicit and implicit ways. Explicit age-related bias is shown in medical policies like age cutoffs for treatment and testing, while implicit bias is hidden in provider and patient attitudes that create barriers in their interactions and so create barriers to care. In my view, implicit ageism is what happened in Sarah's case.

We have seen how bias may cause providers to miss cardiac issues in women, who can have atypical symptom presentations. Older adults also experience negative outcomes when their providers miss diseases that present atypically. Seniors may have no fever with a serious infection, or chest pain may not be present in a heart attack. Instead, nonspecific symptoms such as dizziness, falls, delirium, and decreased appetite are common signs of acute illness in older adults. Health-care providers may fail to make the connection between those nonspecific symptoms and serious disease.

Health-care providers with less geriatric experience may not assess the risk from adverse drug reactions, which significantly increases as patients age. Fortunately, the Beers Criteria® put out by the American

Geriatrics Society (AGS) provides guidelines for potentially inappropriate medications in older adults: medications to avoid in older adults with certain conditions, medications to be used with considerable caution in older adults, medication combinations that may lead to harmful interactions, and a list of medications that should be avoided or dosed differently for those with poor renal function.

Finally, institutional policies may limit access to life-sustaining treatment by rationing care to the aged. For example, costly dialysis and organ transplants during late-stage kidney disease are scrutinized and sometimes denied to older patients. This has been an issue in countries with nationalized health systems like the United Kingdom, although policies have begun to change due to public outcry. In the United States, strictly age-based cut-offs have largely been rejected as explicit age discrimination, in favor of approaches that allocate resources based on the likelihood of a patient to survive hospitalization and live beyond five or ten years. Hospital ethics committees recommend involving the patient, family, and interdisciplinary experts in these complex decisions, with consideration of quality-of-life issues.

The Question of Preventative Screenings

Age has been a factor in the rationing of preventative care. At what age, for example, should we stop authorizing mammograms and colonoscopies for seniors? There are several sets of guidelines to answer this question, but they lack consistency, as you can see from the story of Cora, a vibrant seventy-six-year-old woman new to my practice.

When I met Cora, I was impressed with how proactive she was about her health. She had attended health and wellness workshops and could cite some of the most recent studies published by the Mayo Clinic. She was one of the best health historians I had ever treated, telling me in great detail about all of her conditions and how they were being managed. So I was surprised to hear that she had not had a mammogram in a few years. She told me her last doctor had said she did not need them anymore. He was probably applying guidelines from the United States Preventive Task Force, which states that current evidence is insufficient to assess the balance of benefits and harms of screening mammography in women seventy-five years and older. In contrast, the more aggressive American Cancer Society guidelines recommend that women should continue with mammograms as long as their overall health is good and they have a life expectancy of ten years or more. Cora and I decided to proceed with mammography, and it turned out she did have breast cancer. She was treated and recovered from the disease.

I have another patient who is ninety-three years young and looks like she is seventy-five. Ms. Jackson is self-sufficient, healthy, and on no medications. I would not be surprised if she makes it past one hundred. Against my recommendations, she stopped getting mammograms. One day, she noticed a lump in her breast and came to me for an evaluation. I ordered a mammogram and biopsy, which determined that she had cancer. Fortunately, it was well contained, and with surgery and radiation therapy she is doing quite well and enjoying life.

Both of these cases were judgment calls on my part. With older people, taking a cookie-cutter approach to providing tests and treatment does not work in the best interest of the patient. Guidelines are simply guidelines. I believe we need to approach each patient as an individual and share in decision-making with respect for their own desires.

Older people can have multiple and interrelated conditions. Our treatment goal should be to prevent as many of those conditions as possible and treat the rest with an understanding of the individual patient. That's why selection of a doctor by older patients is very important. Older patients often need to find new doctors because they are moving to retirement communities outside of where their physician practices, or their long-time physician has retired. This means that when an older patient needs their doctor to understand them the most, they may not yet have established a trusting relationship with a new physician.

The importance of geriatric background in an older person's physician is shown in a study of French oncologists' treatment decisions for senior breast cancer patients. The researchers found significant differences in treatment choices depending only on a patient's age. The likelihood of a breast cancer patient undergoing chemotherapy depended on physician specialty and gender, kind of care structure, physicians' beliefs on the age at which patients become "elderly," and their knowledge of geriatric assessments. Some physicians routinely withheld potentially beneficial treatments from senior patients.

Seniors and Mental Health

The World Health Organization (WHO) considers the mental health of our aging population a critical issue. Mental health correlates with the physical health of seniors. The global statistics for mental health and older adults are alarming:

- Mental and neurological disorders account for 6.6 percent of their total disabilities.
- Over 20 percent of adults aged sixty and over suffer from a mental or neurological disorder.
- In the world's older population, dementia and depression affect approximately 5 percent and 7 percent, respectively.
- Anxiety disorders affect 3.8 percent of the older population.
- Substance abuse use problems affect almost 1 percent.
- A quarter of deaths from self-harm are among people aged sixty or above.

For many seniors, growing older is a time of increased stress. They may be experiencing reduced mobility or chronic pain. They are more likely to lose partners, family members, or friends. Retirement may have brought a drop in socioeconomic status. Some have moved away from their close communities for health or financial reasons. These stressors can cause isolation, loneliness, or psychological distress, which impact physical health. Physical conditions can also affect mental health. For example, people with heart disease have higher rates of depression.

One consequence of the COVID pandemic has been the increase in mental health problems due to decreased interaction with other people. For seniors, disrupted personal ties and loneliness impact both their physical and mental health. Isolation reduces access to health care and leads to loneliness, depression, and anxiety.

In their isolation, my patients are increasingly vulnerable to scams. Millions of seniors in this country fall victim to scams at the cost of billions of dollars. Seniors were raised in times when we could be more trusting. They are no less mentally alert or savvy, but they have been raised to believe that people can't just be that bad. The ageist scammers know this, so during times of isolation, these predators prey on lonely seniors. One of my older patients became a victim when her support system just wasn't making enough time for her. She lost a significant amount of money to two scam artists who took advantage of her loneliness by being very friendly and nice to her.

The pandemic has also seen a rise in elder abuse: physical, verbal, psychological, financial, and sexual abuse; abandonment; neglect; and losses of dignity and respect. Prior to the pandemic, evidence indicated that one in six older people had experienced elder abuse. I suspect those numbers have increased. Elder abuse is a form of ageism, where the abusers see the aged as weak and vulnerable.

Another rising number is the incidence of dementia among Americans. Dementia is an impairment in ability to remember, think, or make decisions, which interferes with everyday activities. Alzheimer's disease is the most common type of dementia, with current estimates of 5.6 million people sixty-five and older suffering. Women are nearly two times more likely to be affected by Alzheimer's disease due to women living longer. Minority populations have the fastest growing numbers. By 2060, Hispanics will see a seven-times increase, and cases among African Americans will increase four times over today's estimates. According to the CDC, heart disease and diabetes may account for these differences, as they are more common in Hispanic and African American populations. Lower levels of education, higher rates of poverty, and greater exposure to adversity and discrimination may also increase risk of Alzheimer's disease. This is not something I wanted to hear, already understanding the health disparities faced by minority groups.

The care of people with dementia can be difficult and heartbreaking. For us doctors, communication with dementia patients and their caregivers requires us to maintain respect for the individual before making any assumptions about their age-related cognitive decline. Kathy told me the story of her father. Harry was an avid reader of books on nutrition, and his bible was Adelle Davis's *Let's Eat Right to Keep Fit*, written in 1954. Almost seventy years ago, Davis advocated eating organic fruits, vegetables, and grains and condemned over-processed foods. During the last two years of his life, Harry had dementia. Like many people in his generation, he also had great respect for his doctors, one of whom said to him: "Harry, you can never be too thin." Harry took that as diet advice.

"My father stopped eating," recalled Kathy. "He had no other health conditions and was not on medication. He was functioning well with dementia in the early stages. In familiar situations, the only sign of the disease was his obsession with two passions: the stock market and nutrition. The doctor's words fed into that obsession. We could not get him to eat much of anything, so he became malnourished." Harry collapsed at home and was diagnosed with an irregular heartbeat. While in the hospital, he contracted an infection, which eventually led to his death at age ninety-one.

The doctor tried being compassionate with the family: "Harry had a good long life," he said. That was true, but did the doctor's words encourage a fatal eating disorder in this elderly gentleman with dementia?

When I heard Kathy's story, it made me realize several things. First of all, doctors really need training on how to talk with patients, particularly as they age. Secondly, the doctor was operating from a place of ageism and ableism, seeing ninety-one as being "old enough" and dementia as life-diminishing. And finally, how lucky Harry was to have such a support system in his family.

Seniors and Caregiver Support

Seniors with dementia and other disabilities may need help with the activities of daily living. The age-in-place movement is working to keep seniors in their homes with additional services as needed, but many do move into independent living, assisted living, and nursing homes. No matter where seniors end up living, they often require caregivers, usually family or friends who function as unpaid caregivers. In fact, a 2020 AARP survey found that fifty million people define themselves as taking the role of unpaid caregivers. Ageism and socioeconomic discrimination appear in both the pricing of long-term care and in the lack of respect afforded to seniors and their caregivers.

We talked with Dr. Carolyn A. Brent, who was the primary caregiver for her father for twelve years as his dementia advanced. She took what she learned and became an award-winning author of *The Caregiver's Companion: Caring for Your Loved One Medically, Financially and Emotionally While Caring for Yourself*, as well as a speaker and advocate for family caregivers. "The biggest problem for unpaid caregivers is that society doesn't see it as a job. There is significant bias, and caregivers are often not respected," she said. "Many work full-time in jobs and full-time as unpaid caregivers. There is absolutely no safety net for them. There is no legal protection at work, so caregivers are walking around afraid of losing both their jobs and loved ones."

Carolyn lost a high-paying job because she needed to take care of her father after major brain surgery. "I was asked to choose my father or my job. I chose my father." Now she advocates for laws that would protect unpaid caregivers from job loss.

At one point, Carolyn had to place her father in private assisted care. The costs were astronomical. She was fortunate to have the hard-earned resources to pay, but many people are not able to foot the bill for long-term nursing care. Carolyn advocates for limits to how much care facilities can charge. Care facilities are regulated for their health-care practices, but there is little requirement for financial transparency or pricing caps. As a primary physician, I have seen many of my patients faced with the impossibly high cost of assisted living and nursing homes. No matter how much money they have saved, who can afford ten thousand dollars per month? The prices are simply ridiculous. And, contrary to many people's belief, Medicare does not cover long-term care. That's another reason why the needed caregiving tasks end up in the hands of unpaid family.

Carolyn said two of the most important lessons she learned as an unpaid caregiver were that knowledge is power and self-care is essential. "Caregivers need to become mini doctors. They need to look at the evidence-based research in order to advocate for the people they are taking care of. They need to know their loved one's medical history inside and out. I recommend creating a binder of all records to take with you to any health-care provider." Going in to face the health-care system as an advocate for her vulnerable father, knowing that she would face ageism and lack of respect for her as a caregiver, Carolyn armed herself with knowledge and self-confidence.

Carolyn is an African American woman. I am not surprised that she was devoted to the personal caregiving of her father. I often see Black women accompanying my patients, which is not surprising since women remain the primary source of caregiving. But I also see many Black men accompany their wives, mothers, sisters, and aunties to office visits, and several are the primary caregiver of a relative. I have also seen this with my Asian American patients. I have observed that African American, Hispanic, and Asian American cultures seem to provide more caregiving to older family members. My White patients usually come alone or with a paid caregiver. One ninety-year-old White patient is accompanied by her son, but he acts so begrudging of the time he spends with his mother that my patient is always anxious and nervous. I feel bad for her. But we need scientific research to validate my anecdotal observations about culture and caregiving. We need to be able to provide support systems for non-paid caregivers based on cultural differences, without making assumptions based on how our own culture treats the aged.

Ageism comes up during end-of-life decisions for patients, families, and providers. Again, it comes down to respect for the individual patient's wishes. Families can get in the way of the patient's decision-making because of their own attitudes toward aging, their fears, and anticipated loss. Deciding to decline treatment when faced with a terminal illness or accident is painful for all involved. But, at the end of the day, I firmly believe in honoring a patient's desires based on how they see the quality of their life. To choose a natural death, allowing a person to decide when enough is enough, is a right all of us should have. On the other hand, as a provider, I would not presume to withhold life-sustaining treatment just because a patient is advanced in age. Among medical providers, I think I am rare in this attitude.

Removing Ageism from Health Care

If we are going to remove ageism from health care, we need to change our attitudes about seniors. This quote from Dr. Sharon Inouye, internationally recognized leader in geriatric medicine and aging research, resonates with me: "Undervaluing older adults endangers us all. In the context of health care, older adults are often viewed as an economic burden on resources; however, the reality is that older adults are the bedrock and foundation upon which our society is built, based on their past, current, and future contributions to society and the economy."

When we view older adults as invisible, a burden, or physically and mentally unfit, we reinforce the societal, interpersonal, and internalized biases that diminish the quality of life for the bedrock of our society. We need to act on recommendations from anti-ageist experts:

- Provide just and equitable access to life-sustaining treatments and procedures.
- Expand the number of geriatric specialists.
- Require rotations in geriatrics in medical schools, as they are required in pediatrics.
- Add older patients to clinical trials to determine safe dosage and treatment.
- Take a holistic approach to aging, recognizing the complex emotional, mental, and physical changes as people age.
- Support unpaid caregivers in the workplace and at home.

Most important, we must honor and respect those who go before us. No matter what our roles, backgrounds, or status, we are all human beings who one day will be in the same spot as those who are older than us. Just as we embrace a newborn with pride and wonder, we need to embrace our grandmas and grandpas, aunts and uncles, and dear older friends with that same pride and wonder. I try to visit my aunt Jane often. Sometimes it is to help her out, but most often I want to experience this amazing woman who I am so lucky to have in my life. We all have Aunt Janes who can enrich our lives even more than we enrich theirs.

Kathy experiences this enrichment across the generations every day. She lives in a multigenerational household with her son and two grandchildren, who moved in after she was widowed. Later, she was blessed when her new husband joined the household. She will tell you that it's great having young people around to help with the big old house, but that's just an incidental benefit. The real benefit is that she gets to live in her own personal Blue Zone, where she has a life filled with purpose and connection. She is never lonely and finds intense happiness being involved in her grandchildren's lives; she knows what music they like, and occasionally holds dance parties or beats them in Uno. Most important, she knows ageism will never occur to her son's or grandchildren's minds because they find as much joy in her as she does in them.

CHAPTER 10

How We Devalue
People with Disabilities

I HAVE EXPERIENCED THE MOST personal growth as a physician from my most vulnerable patients: patients with physical or intellectual disabilities. When I first started, I knew my new Comprehensive Women's Health practice would attract more health-conscious women. After all, healthy patients who take a proactive role in their health are the easiest to treat. But I have grown insight, wisdom, and empathy from working with my more "complex" patients: those with disabilities.

I have realized how often we devalue people with disabilities instead of seeing the gifts they bring. I am now aware of *ableism*, the discrimination and social prejudice against people with disabilities or people who are perceived to be disabled. This ism characterizes people with disabilities as *inferior* to the non-disabled. As a Black woman, I can relate to being treated as inferior, but a person with disabilities faces another set of obstacles. My patients are a constant source of learning for me in how to be a better doctor and a better person.

My patients have reminded me of the need to advocate for yourself. Mary is a patient who has a cognitive disability, the result of a brain tumor as a young adult. The tumor required surgical removal and left her with a seizure disorder and cognitive deficits. Her very slurred speech makes her difficult to understand. But Mary comes to her appointments with a notepad of questions and concerns, is proactive about her health, and always lets me know how much she appreciates the time I spend with her. Recently, she shared that she had to change specialists due to insurance coverage, and the new doctor did not treat her as well. "He didn't even look at me. I never want to go back to him," she said. We worked together to find another specialist who will treat her with the attention she deserves. Mary knew how to stand up for herself and seek help when she felt shortchanged in her health care.

My experience with another patient reminded me to be respectful of individual choices. Susan was a successful medical professional prior to a traumatic brain injury in her thirties. That loss of independence put her in a group home. Sometimes at her medical visits she would appear sad and grumpy. After getting her to open up about her frustrations, I learned that Mary was upset that she was not allowed to smoke at the group home. Of course, I had to remind her of smoking's damage to her health, but she finally told me, "I know all that, but it's *my* choice." I finally heard and respected her individual choice, so I asked the group home to allow Susan to go outside to smoke a few times a day. Sure, it still bothers me that she smokes, but it is her choice. Having lost some independence living in the group home, her choice to smoke is one thing she feels she can control.

I have also learned from my patients that ableism can be very subtle. Shanice was born with severe cognitive deficits and has the mental functioning of a child. Her childhood doctors predicted her life expectancy would be short. She has proved those doctors wrong by outliving many of them. On one of her visits, I realized that I had failed to recommend her for a colonoscopy, even though she met the age criteria. My ableist bias had created a blind spot to Shanice's needs. Since then, I have made sure to follow all the age-appropriate screening recommendations for Shanice. She may be cognitively disabled, but she is otherwise a healthy adult with a normal life expectancy.

Living with Disabilities in America

Disability is not rare. Sixty-one million adults in the United States live with one. That means that 26 percent, one in four adults, have at least one disability in mobility, cognition, or impaired sight or hearing. Older adults, women, and minorities are more likely to have disabilities. Two in five adults over sixty-five, one in four women, and two in five American Indians and Alaska Natives live with disabilities.

People with disabilities are more likely to have health risk factors such as smoking or obesity. Almost 12 percent have heart disease, compared to 4 percent of Americans without disabilities, and 16 percent have diabetes compared to 7 percent without disabilities. Their access to health care is limited: One in three adults with disabilities aged eighteen to forty-four do not have a primary provider and have unmet health-care needs because of cost and transportation challenges. One in four adults with disabilities aged forty-five to sixty-four does not have routine checkups.

There are lots of reasons for these inequities—socioeconomic factors, lack of caregiver support, and societal bias, but we physicians have also contributed to the problem. In a survey of 714 practicing physicians nationwide, 82 percent reported that they believed people with a disability have a worse quality of life than non-disabled people. Only 41 percent of physicians were very confident in their ability to provide the same quality of care to patients with a disability. Only 56 percent strongly agreed that they welcomed patients with a disability into their practices. But less than 20 percent strongly agreed that the health-care system often treats these patients unfairly. The researchers concluded, "More than thirty years after the Americans with Disabilities Act of 1990 was enacted, these findings about physicians' perceptions of this population raise questions about ensuring equitable care to people with a disability. Potentially biased views among physicians could contribute to persistent health-care disparities affecting people with disability."

The "Quality of Life" Bias

The most powerful statistic from that survey of physicians was that *82 percent reported that individuals with significant disabilities have worse quality of life than individuals without disabilities.* These doctors are making an unfounded generalization about these individuals. Their judgments of poor quality of life could lead them to believe that people with disabilities' lives are inferior, and then to assume that they are an inferior group of people. Such thinking is the source of ableism and a dangerous mindset for doctors: We are the decision-makers about who gets which medical treatment and who does not. We health-care providers must constantly weigh hard ethical questions about treatment and quality of life, particularly with very sick patients or in end-of-life cases. That is the nature of our profession. However, we cannot base our decisions on an assumption that an individual with disabilities has a less valuable life.

We saw an extreme example of devaluation in Nazi Germany. Most of us know about the six million Jews who were murdered under Hitler, but fewer are aware that more than two hundred thousand people with physical and mental disabilities were also systematically killed. Nazism's T-4 program saw them as genetically impure, useless to society, and unworthy of life. Many German doctors participated in this atrocity by reviewing medical files to determine who should live and who should die. Adults with disabilities were sent to gas chambers; children and infants with disabilities were given lethal injections or starved to death.

Kathy recalls visiting the Holocaust Museum in Washington, DC, with Mark, a friend who was born with congenital hip disease, has had four hip replacements, and walks with a cane. "Mark and I looked at each other and realized that both of us would have died if we had lived in Nazi Germany. I am Jewish, and he is an individual with disabilities. We would not have had a chance."

But prejudice against people with disabilities is not just a thing of the past. According to the United Nations, mortality for children with disabilities may be as high as 80 percent, and in some cases children with disabilities are being intentionally "weeded out." Individuals with disabilities are more likely to be victims of violence or rape and less likely to obtain police intervention and legal protection. This is not just a Third World problem. It's happening right here in the United States. Violent crimes against individuals with disabilities are on the rise in our country, particularly against women. Individuals with disabilities are four to ten times more likely to become victims of violence, abuse, or neglect than individuals without disabilities. Children with disabilities are more than twice as likely to be physically or sexually abused as children without disabilities.

There are laws in the United States to protect people with disabilities, but if the health-care system assumes that quality and value of life are based solely on being "able," patients can be dismissed from quality care. Patients are further endangered if their disability impedes their ability to communicate their treatment preferences and quality of life desires. Life-and-death decisions are made for them without consultation with the patient.

One dramatic example of this occurred in a Texas hospital, where Michael Hickson died after being admitted from a nursing home with COVID. Three years before, the forty-six-year-old Black, college-educated father of five children had suffered cardiac arrest, with loss of oxygen leaving him brain injured, blind, and with quadriplegia. Though he had trouble moving and talking, he was still involved in his children's lives. His wife, Melissa, posted YouTube videos of the family gathered around Michael's bed, talking and singing.

At the hospital, Michael quickly deteriorated. His health team decided to deny potentially life-saving care and withhold nutrition and hydration. He was moved from the ICU to hospice care. His wife questioned the decision. The hospital was not yet at the point of having to ration care due to COVID overload. They just denied her husband care. She posted a recording of her conversation with the doctor:

Doctor: The decision is: Do we want to be extremely aggressive with his care or do we feel like this would be futile? As of right now, his quality of life—he doesn't have much of one.

Melissa Hickson: What do you mean? Because he's paralyzed with a brain injury, he doesn't have quality of life?

Doctor: Correct.

The disability community reacted with anger. The National Council on Disability (NCD) issued a statement: "NCD denounces this denial of life-saving care. The presence of a disability does not lessen a person's value, nor should it warrant a person's abandonment by the medical facilities they rely on for care...."

But there is even more to the story. Neither Melissa nor her husband had made the decision to discontinue treatment. The sign-off was made by his medical guardian, an eldercare agency. According to an NPR report, prior to COVID, a Texas probate court had replaced Melissa as her husband's guardian after she had disagreed with decisions made by a previous hospital. As the NPR article reported, "It's not unusual for caregivers and medical staff to fight. It's unusual, though, that a probate court would step in."

Melissa is adamant that her husband would have wanted treatment if he had been asked. "He would say, 'I want to live. I love my family and my children and they're the most important things to me.' He would probably say that's the reason for the past three years I have fought to survive."

Caregiving for People with Disabilities

One of my first patients, Susie, was paralyzed from the waist down due to a severe neurological disorder. She was fortunate to have the best husband on earth, Mike, who accompanied her to every doctor's appointment. He was intimately familiar with her health and took very good care of his wife. A highly educated corporate executive, he was so attentive that I wondered how he could also manage a busy career. One day I asked him, "Now, I know Susie is doing well, but how are *you* doing? I know that caregiving can take a toll on your health." He confidently replied, "Oh, my doctor says I'm healthy as a horse!"

A year later, Mike was diagnosed with an aggressive cancer and died. We were all devastated, but no one more than Susie, who went into a deep depression. She had lost not only the love of her life but also her dedicated caregiver. No family member was willing or able to step into the huge shoes that Mike left. Susie's care suffered, and she finally had to move from their home to an assisted living facility. Susie and Mike were lucky to have the financial resources to afford it. She was treated well there, but not nearly as well as with Mike. She died about a year after Mike, and I am sure that the depression that followed his death played a role in her untimely passing.

Finding quality care can be a major issue for individuals with disabilities. Many of my patients do not have the family support or financial means to support themselves or to afford decent caregiving services. Good home caregivers are expensive and in high demand. Some experts predict a national shortage of 151,000 caregivers by 2030 and a 355,000-caregiver shortfall by 2040 as our population ages. Family and friends sometimes take on the responsibility, but the needed care can be too difficult or involved for untrained caregivers. Without family support, individuals with disabilities must find skilled, affordable paid home care, or resort to a long-term care facility.

I am awestruck by the loving and respectful care from both unpaid and paid caregivers. They are heroic, though caregiver burnout and stress take a toll. We have recently become more aware of the need to provide respite care and caregiver self-care training. The news runs an occasional sensational story of abuse or neglect by a bad-apple caregiver, but I believe most caregivers rise to the challenges of this difficult and stressful job.

The relationships among patients with disabilities, their caregivers, and their doctors are delicate and complex. I have learned a great deal about my patients when I've taken the time to see and listen to *them* instead of just addressing their caregivers. Patients with disabilities have complicated health histories, they may be on many medications, and they may have several specialists that we primaries need to coordinate with. The patients' communication impairments might require more time to listen and understand them, so we need to build in more time for their appointments, look our patients in the eye, listen to them, and then coordinate closely with the caregivers.

Primary doctors often have a more stable role in a patient's life than their paid caregivers, whose job turnover is high. We must know our patients' baselines so we can monitor for any change in their condition. We can alert their caregivers to signs of change and train new caregivers in care skills tailored to the patient's needs. We need to discuss the sensitive but essential issues of hygiene, toileting, and sexuality. Out of respect for the patient, we should know what they are comfortable talking about in front of their caregiver.

Linda has taught me a lot about the patient-caregiver relationship. She lives in a group home for people with traumatic brain injuries, several of whom are my patients. Linda is a forty-year-old woman who experienced a traumatic brain injury in her twenties, leaving her neurologically impaired. She cannot walk unassisted, has difficulty speaking, and is hearing impaired, but receives amazing support from both her family and the caregivers at the group home. Linda recently had a fall that resulted in a fracture. She went to the ER, where the doctors immediately suspected abuse and started interrogating her caregivers. Linda politely interjected, "No, it wasn't their fault. I'm just really clumsy." During our own visits, she does not hesitate to interrupt me when I aim my explanation of a treatment plan at her caregivers. "Excuse me, what is it that you are recommending?" she will ask, reminding me to look directly at her so she can read my lips. Linda keeps me on my toes, and I am grateful that she does.

More Alike Than Different

The worst mistake of the ableist is their belief that people with disabilities are less-than or inferior to the rest of us. But think of Stephen Hawking, the world-famous theoretical physicist and cosmologist, who from age thirty was paralyzed with motor neuron disorder (amyotrophic lateral sclerosis, or ALS) but made his greatest contributions to his field after the onset of his disability. Think of Beethoven, who could not hear a note when he wrote the Ninth Symphony, one of the most important classical pieces of all time. Think how our hearts have been lifted by the voices of Stevie Wonder and Andrea Bocelli, both of whom are blind, and Teddy Pendergrass, who suffered from quadriplegia.

But it is the stories of extraordinary "ordinary" people that are most moving. Kathy has worked with several authors with mental and intellectual disabilities and felt as privileged working with them as I have in helping my patients. She has learned important lessons from her authors. The first lesson was in bravery: Eric Weaver is a retired police sergeant whose battles against disabling depression and PTSD brought him to the brink of suicide several times. Eric channeled his own suffering into creating a training program to destigmatize mental illness in the police force. His powerful and candid book is called *Overcoming the Darkness: Shining Light on Mental Illness, Trauma and Suicide in Law Enforcement.*

Kathy's second lesson was that we are *More Alike Than Different,* which is the title of David Egan's memoir of his life with Down syndrome. David has become a global advocate for seeing the similarities among people regardless of our so-called "abilities." He has made sure that people never saw him as "inferior." His words move me: "In my life, I have learned that the barriers of low expectations aren't real. In a way, they mark the limits of imagination. If someone hasn't seen or heard of someone doing something, maybe they think it can't be done. . . ."

Erasing Ableism from Health Care

While we may be seeing decreased race and gender discrimination in America, our health-care system is still riddled with ableism. This is particularly disturbing for us in medicine, since the medical field is given the power, often the legal power, to determine who is disabled, why, and what their potential may be. We often make these decisions based on our assessment of a person's quality of life, yet studies have consistently shown that health-care professionals underestimate the quality of life of people with disabilities.

So how do we get health-care providers to value people with disabilities? Start with their medical training: Include the perspectives of real people with disabilities in medical school classes. Familiarize students with the experience of people who live routinely with feeding tubes, respirators, and assistive technology. Show students that these people's lives are just another form of normal.

That is just the beginning. Andrés J. Gallegos, who chairs the National Council of Disability and advises the president, Congress, and federal agencies on national disability policy writes: "Explicit and implicit discriminatory bias within the health-care professions represent an insidious virus against which people with disabilities have been fighting for decades. The breadth of the problem is already clear and does not warrant more research.... I believe we must respond collectively to address the discriminatory bias."

Gallegos recommends four actions. The first is to include disability-focused cultural competency courses in all health-care professional schools. Few medical schools currently include such a curriculum. Secondly, he wants state legislation to require care facilities to use an independent, due-process mechanism for mediating and deciding medical futility disputes. Medical futility refers to interventions that are judged unlikely to produce any significant benefit for the patient. Third, Gallegos wants an alternative to the use of "quality-adjusted life years" (QALYs) to determine the value of health outcomes. Some

Medicaid programs and an increasing number of private health insurers, government agencies, and health economists use QALYs as the formula to secure cost savings. Finally, he advocates strengthening existing federal nondiscrimination laws and engaging in more robust enforcement.

I'll leave you with one last thought. An individual can belong simultaneously to several groups that face bias, and that is often true of individuals with disabilities. Black adults are more likely to have disabilities than White adults. Women are more likely to have disabilities than men. Older people are more likely to have disabilities than younger people. Adults with disabilities are more likely to be obese than adults without a disability. So if you are an older, obese, Black woman with disabilities, you are probably being dismissed by our health-care system, and you may never know which factor was the reason why. Probably more than one.

CHAPTER 11

Dealing with the Shame of Obesity

S AN AFRICAN AMERICAN WOMAN who has experienced medical racism, I was surprised to find out that no topic in our bias survey elicited more comments than weight. Many people had a story to tell about feeling shamed or dismissed when seeing a health-care provider. In fact, 34 percent said they have been treated differently by a medical professional because of their body type.

As a doctor, I know that obesity can cause or exacerbate many medical conditions. The risks of type 2 diabetes, coronary heart disease, stroke, sleep apnea, osteoarthritis, and some types of cancers are all increased when people are obese. And it is likely that our patients will be overweight or obese: More than two thirds of Americans fall into one of those two categories, and fifteen million are diagnosed as morbidly obese.

That means that most people who walk into a doctor's office, urgent care, or hospital are going to have a "weight problem." So how will we react? Will we judge them? Will our own biases and issues with weight affect how we treat them? Our survey showed that patients feel we health-care providers are not doing a great job.

Some of those stories related to misdiagnosis since obesity is perceived as the cause:

Was having symptoms of dizziness and felt tired all the time. He immediately told me to change my diet and gave me a sermon about sugars and obesity. I explained I have been eating more healthily and these feelings were different. My doctor reiterated his opinion of obesity. Not long after, I had a TIA (ministroke). I changed doctors, and even though he wouldn't say anything against what the previous doctor said [about] obesity [being] a contributing factor, he actually listened. We had a conversation and ordered additional testing and developed a plan of treatment [when] he found out that I had leukemia.

I went to an urgent care for back pain and the provider didn't want to give me anything. He said I was fat. I went to my own doctor later, got X-rays, and found out I had arthritis from a past back injury.

I was experiencing significant foot pain. I finally went to a podiatrist. She was smart, young, and 100 percent convinced that the foot pain was a result of my weight. She dismissed any questions I had and suggested that I perform foot stretches. The pain continued and gradually increased. After consulting a different doctor, realized the foot was broken in two places, requiring surgery for repair.

Other stories talked about the attitude of health-care providers, specifically about losing weight:

Went for post-op visit after hysterectomy for uterine cancer. Had already been advised by surgeon that I should work on losing weight due to increased production of estrogen in fat cells. I was dieting and had lost fourteen pounds in eight weeks, which is the rate the doctor had advised. The physician assistant grimaced when she uncovered my body to do the exam. She started to lecture me about needing to lose weight. I asked her if she had even looked at my chart or noticed I was losing weight. She just went back to lecturing me. I informed her that I would be switching to my family doctor for all further cancer surveillance exams. I had a good talk with my family doc about the encounter with the PA. She was quite indignant that I had been treated so disrespectfully and was very happy to provide me follow-up care.

I was pregnant with my second child and the doctor at the OB-GYN practice I was using was lecturing me about gaining as little weight as possible (I had not gained an inordinate amount of weight). However, pregnancy is not an easy time to keep one's weight down because one is always hungry! Because this doctor weighed 250–300 pounds, I told him I thought anyone his size had no business telling me I needed to keep my weight down. That ended the conversation. I didn't see him again for quite a while, but when I did, interestingly enough, he had lost a substantial amount of weight. Touché, Doc! I was only nineteen years old at the time.

I met with a doctor to get a second opinion about my fibroids. Instead of listening to my concerns, she proceeds to tell me I am overweight. She didn't offer any assistance in helping me figure out what other options I had outside of a hysterectomy. I felt judged and ridiculed, especially since I was working on weight loss and had lost weight prior to seeing her. It was clear to me she didn't take the time to even read over my chart. She was rude and didn't have a good bedside manner. I submitted a complaint but doubt anything was done about it.

Sometimes I feel dismissed from new doctors who only
want to focus on my weight. I've been dealing with this since
I [was] six years old. I only had a few doctors [who] understood what I was dealing with and treated me, rather than
just telling me to lose weight.

My current doctor does listen to me but sometimes other
doctors/PAs who don't know me, I feel, may make assumptions because of my weight.

My ob-gyn basically said I had gotten fat since my last visit.
I had gained [the] freshmen twenty and didn't need to hear
it from him!

Still other complaints related to assigning blame to the patient:

I had taken a fall in a restaurant. There was a piece of food
left on the tile floor. I did not see it and when my foot made
contact, I slipped and fell. The doctor said I hurt myself not
so much because of the fall itself but because of my body
size. I was absolutely shocked.

Overweight older woman. Everything is the result of overweight and I should not complain. Docs don't understand
or believe my genetic diagnosis (Ehlers-Danlos syndrome,
which affects connective tissue, primarily the skin, joints,
and blood vessel walls).

My medical record indicates I am morbidly obese. This despite being active, eating healthy, don't smoke. I wear an
Apple Watch and can download certain activity/medical
records to prove I am making an earnest attempt in staying
healthy. And I don't have high blood pressure or diabetes!

She relates everything back to my weight, not the symptoms or underlying condition. I now use a DO (Doctor of Osteopathic Medicine), which is MUCH better than my experiences with a MD.

I'm an RN and have faced discrimination in health care for obesity all my life. Most of the time, an MD doesn't even touch me during an "exam." Here's a current example: Despite having scheduled a THR (total hip replacement) for the end of April, when I [was] sent to pre-op on 4/5, MD said he was "rethinking" the surgery because he recently had two obese patients develop infections. I have no risk factors for infection/complication or history of infection with any surgery. He kept looking at the hip X-ray and saying, "That hip is terrible" and then saying he didn't want to move forward. I told him I have no information on the medical status of the other patients or who was practicing what prevention techniques; that it was cruel to deny my surgery when he could see my level of suffering. Unfortunately, a-fib was identified on EKG, so he has a reprieve for now.

I don't know how those stories make you feel, but they hurt my heart. There's a lot of pain and anger there. Clearly, shaming or dismissal for weight occurs across medical specialties, conditions, and types of health-care providers. Age and gender do not seem to matter.

I don't believe that our survey was an anomaly. In fact, a *New York Times* article, "Why Do Obese Patients Get Worse Care? Many Doctors Don't See Past the Fat," received more than twelve hundred online comments, and people primarily shared negative experiences. While the article did not examine the psychological effects of fat-shaming by doctors, it did cite research that doctors who focus on a patient's weight spend less time with them, order fewer diagnostic tests, and more often prescribe lifestyle changes instead of medication, compared to their patients of normal weight.

Societal Bias against Obesity

Bias against overweight and obese people in our country is rampant. Society is cruel to people, particularly girls and women if they are outside of "normal" body types. Disturbing recent reports show the effects of social-media body-shaming on young people, particularly girls, linking it to anxiety, depression, and even suicide among teenagers. Bias against "fat" is behind job discrimination, relationship problems, and bullying in schools.

Weight is on many of our minds. My co-author, Kathy, looks to advice columns in popular magazines for insights into the minds of the public. For six months she tracked "Dear Abby," "Ask Amy," "Dear Prudence," and *People Magazine*'s advice column and found that on average, in fourteen articles or letters per week writers expressed pain about being overweight or celebrated weight loss. The weight issue came up more than any other topic.

In one advice column, a young mother reported that she was fifteen pounds overweight and very active, exercising five days a week, but had a thyroid condition that made it hard for her to lose weight. Her husband constantly hounded and ridiculed her about her weight. She was distraught and wanted to know how to get him to back off. Nothing she said or did made a difference to him. The advice columnist responded that the husband was vicious, insensitive, and fatphobic. She suggested the woman seek therapy to figure out why she would remain married to someone who intentionally hurt her. Kathy and I both thought this was good advice.

While explicit bias directed at race, gender, age, or disabilities is now seen as wrong in our society, explicit bias against the obese is still tolerated. Laws do not protect against discrimination based on body size. The movements against fat-shaming and for body positivity are working for change, but the change is slow. Society has acknowledged that people don't have a choice about their race, gender, age, or physical and mental disabilities, but being overweight or obese is viewed as the result of laziness and lack of discipline. Society has accepted that conditions like alcoholism and drug addiction are diseases largely beyond the patient's control, but does not label obesity in the same way, even though doctors do chart it as a disease.

It is not surprising that health-care providers mirror society's lack of compassion for the obese. One national study of almost five thousand first-year medical students found that they exhibited implicit (74 percent) and explicit (67 percent) weight bias. Implicit weight bias scores were comparable to reported bias against racial minorities. Explicit attitudes were more negative toward obese people than toward other groups. With health-care providers' attitudes like this, no wonder the patient experience is so difficult for so many.

The Patient Experience and Responsibility

On top of their negative attitude, health-care professionals often do not have the equipment to treat obese patients with dignity. The patients are subject to embarrassment when blood pressure cuffs and gowns don't fit. They may have difficulty getting up and down from examining tables. Medical office scales may not measure beyond 250 pounds, sending the obese patient to a freight scale. MRI and CT scanners are too small for some patients. Hospital beds are too small. The obese patient is repeatedly humiliated in the health-care system.

About that scale ... That five-letter word puts fear in the hearts of so many. Few patients want to get on a scale at the doctor's office. I get it. As a person who has also struggled with weight gain over the years, I hate getting on a scale. Unfortunately, few patients understand that getting their weight is an essential part of our full medical examination. Just like blood pressure, temperature, respiratory rate, and pulse, we consider your weight among the vital signs. Weight loss or gain can be indicators of potential health issues. We should check all your vitals at every visit. Just imagine if you came into a doctor's office for knee pain, but we didn't take your blood pressure. The next day you have a stroke. We missed finding hypertension, one of the "silent killers." Weighing you is the same as taking your blood pressure: Weight gain or loss can be a sign of many of these silent killers. We doctors need to know what is going on inside you, and weight change is one indicator of your health.

Getting weighed at the doctor's office is also a reality check. Some people have such acute scale avoidance at home that the only time they're weighed is there at the doctor's office. When people gain weight, it's usually in small increments. We may not be aware of how much we've gained or lost. Often when the weight goes up, so does cholesterol and blood sugar. But without a medical checkup, including weight, those conditions might remain hidden. When people lose weight, cholesterol, pre-diabetes, and diabetes numbers usually get better. Though you may be reluctant to get on that scale, knowing your weight is important to your overall health.

Our problem is how we health-care providers talk to patients about weight. Just telling them, "You need to lose weight" assumes that the fat patient doesn't know this already. Too often our anti-weight bias makes us treat the fat patient as stupid. We can't assume lack of intelligence from a patient's lifestyle choices. It would be just as naïve for us to assume that smokers don't understand that smoking is harmful to their health. A person would have to live in a cave not to know that it's bad for them. We are not helping the patient by bluntly reminding them.

Weight is a hot button for many people, and visits to doctors' offices often push that button. Some patients are wary of seeking medical care if a past doctor has attributed all their health problems to obesity without a thorough diagnostic process or has prescribed weight loss as a cure for all ills. The patient assumes, based on previous experiences, that they will be blamed or dismissed. Because of that experience of being stigmatized, humiliated, and shamed for their weight, the patient can have serious mental and physical health consequences. The patient might stop going to doctors altogether.

I do believe, however, that patients must also take responsibility when it comes to working to maintain a healthy weight. I have talked quite a lot about patients ignoring a doctor's diagnosis and treatment recommendations or turning to Dr. Google for advice instead of evidence-based research. Weight loss is primary area where I see patients either not understanding or not wanting to understand the proven consequences of obesity. Every single piece of evidence points to heart disease, type 2 diabetes, some cancers, arthritis, and more being connecting to what you put in your body and how you move. Instead, my patients will opt for medication to lower sugar, blood pressure, and cholesterol. Then some even say they have good numbers. Yes, they have good numbers because the medication is working. But why medicate if just taking off a small percentage of weight would make those numbers go down. And what I really don't get is why people don't understand that getting to a healthy weight is all about moving more and eating better. Instead, people are always looking for something else—a better cure. And they are willing to pay for it. The weight-loss industry is HUGE. In 2019, it was $78 billion annually in the United States alone. There are literally thousands of diets, products, and plans that will all promise weight loss. Some are legit; most are not. Some are even dangerous.

My own prescription to my patients is clear. Every month, change one habit that contributes to weight gain. Too many soft drinks? Get rid of them for a month. No exercise? Walk for a month. Donuts every day? Say goodbye for a month. Eating out? Cook for a month. Making these changes will give you lasting beneficial health habits. Is this idea remarkable? No. In fact, I suspect most primary doctors would say, "Just do it."

The Health Consequences of Weight Stigma

Research has found that people with obesity use health-care services less. Weight bias is a major barrier to their engaging with health-care providers, pointing to several factors that discouraged patient engagement with primary care health professionals: contemptuous, patronizing, or disrespectful treatment; ambivalence; attribution of all health issues to excess weight; assumptions about weight gain; expectation of differential health-care treatment; low trust and poor communication.

One major result of weight bias is psychological distress. Research shows that individuals who identify as being overweight or obese have internalized weight stigma as depression, anxiety, and stress. Weight bias internalization (WBI) occurs when people apply negative weight stereotypes to themselves, interfering with their relationships with parents, spouses, friends, teachers, and health-care providers. The damaging effects of WBI include self-shaming, negative weight-related attitudes, and self-stereotyping. WBI can also result in weight gain and disordered eating. "Epidemiologic and experimental evidence of the harms of WBI is mounting, including poorer self-reported health and health-related quality of life, binge eating, and maladaptive health behaviors."

Dr. Rebecca L. Pearl, adjunct assistant professor of psychiatry and director of the University of Florida Body Image and Stigma (BIAS) Lab, has done extensive research on WBI. Her work explores the biological, social, and structural ways that WBI affects health and what perpetuates or prevents weight stigma. In a news article about her work, Dr. Pearl said, "There is a common misconception that stigma might help motivate individuals with obesity to lose weight and improve their health. We are finding it has quite the opposite effect. When people feel shamed because of their weight, they are more likely to avoid exercise and consume more calories to cope with this stress."

In the study, the researchers discovered a significant relationship between internalizing weight bias and being diagnosed with metabolic syndrome. Metabolic syndrome is a cluster of conditions including increased blood pressure, high blood sugar, excess body fat around the waist, and abnormal cholesterol or triglyceride levels. Metabolic syndrome increases your risk of heart disease, stroke, and type 2 diabetes. Her co-author, Dr. Tom Wadden, professor of psychology in psychiatry at the University of Pennsylvania Perelman School of Medicine and Director of Penn Center for Weight and Eating Disorders, added: "Providers can play a critical role in decreasing this internalization by treating patients with respect, discussing weight with sensitivity and without judgment, and giving support and encouragement to patients who struggle with weight management—behaviors everyone should display when interacting with people with obesity."

Taking Judgment out of the Equation

Research on weight bias in health care recommends better medical communication training. Health-care providers need to understand that when they address patients with negative weight bias, they can unintentionally drive weight gain and cause poorer health. More compassionate and knowledgeable health-care providers would deliver better care to obese patients.

Medical training is a good start, but I think we need to go beyond that. Laws and regulations against discrimination in the workplace were vital steps in addressing racism. Protection of people with disabilities added accountability to caregivers to reduce mistreatment and equalized public accessibility. Society at large needs to add the bias against obesity to its list of -isms to be outlawed. But let's just start with us health-care providers. We have assumed that by shaming obese people we will help them achieve weight loss, but evidence now shows that fat-shaming has the opposite effect. In addition, we can cause emotional and mental stress that brings harm to those patients' health.

Shaming ends when judgment ends. As health-care providers, it may be difficult for us to withhold judgment on people we may think are "unworthy" of our care and services because they seem to disregard their own health. A diabetic who is noncompliant with their medication. A smoker. A person with high blood pressure who eats too much salt. But the ethical standard of our profession requires us to resist the temptation to judge.

Earlier, I told you about admiring my mentor doctors who gave nonjudgmental care of criminal suspects in the hospital and my learning from my grandmother's compassionate care of inmates in prison. If we can care nonjudgmentally for mass murders and criminals, then surely we can care for others that way. We need to recheck our ethical standards and make sure we understand our role as professionals. We must see our patients without judgment, understanding the vulnerability that each of them brings into the health-care environment. And then we must take sensitive, respectful care of that vulnerable patient.

This lesson was brought home to me by a patient I'll call Ella. Ella called our office to ask us to refill a prescription for prednisone because her legs were swollen. She was categorized as a high-risk patient because of her frequent ER visits. Reviewing her chart, I realized that for two years she had only had video visits with our office, none in person. During her last video visit she hadn't even appeared on camera. I called and told her she needed to come in person so we could check her vitals and do some diagnostic testing before refilling her prednisone. She was very resistant, insisting that since the ER had recently discharged her to home, there was no need for another doctor visit. And she admitted that before, when she was four hundred pounds, it had been easier for her to get around. Now that she was over five hundred pounds, it was too difficult for her to come into the office.

I reassured her that our office was a no-judgment zone, and she need not worry about us commenting on her weight gain. Again, she pushed back, saying that she was very aware of her weight, wasn't worried about it, and was thinking of having bariatric surgery. She also reiterated that the hospital had said she was fine. I explained that just because the hospital had said she was not having a heart attack at that moment did not mean she was fine. I worried that she had a false sense that she was okay. Once again I asked her to come in so we could do some preventative care. She still refused and insisted that the medication refill was all she needed. Prednisone had worked on her leg swelling before and would work again. She insisted that she had no concerns about how she would be viewed; she just had trouble getting around these days. I really thought both factors were involved, but that thought didn't really matter to the practical need of the moment. What mattered was that she must be seen. I admitted to myself that my argument was not going to sway her and arranged for a home visit. Was that my ideal solution? Absolutely not. Was it difficult to see my patient so resistant to getting the help she needed? Definitely. But I needed to individualize my care of this patient to get the job done.

Fortunately, I have a code of ethics that I use as my touchstone: the Hippocratic oath. When I face a patient who doesn't fit the norm of size or compliance, this line stands out for me: *I will remember that I remain a member of society, with special obligations to all my fellow human beings, those sound of mind and body as well as the infirm.* Remembering this, I go forward in my quest to treat all my patients as individual human beings, without judgment or shame. I dream of a day when the entire health-care system can become a sincere, no-judgment zone.

PART 3

Complex Challenges to Our Health-Care System

Although the world is full of suffering, it is full also of the overcoming of it.

— HELEN KELLER

CHAPTER 12

Social Determinants of Health

SOCIAL DETERMINANTS OF HEALTH (SDOH) sounds like a pretty important academic term. It is. Researchers, educators, and policy makers across disciplines use SDOH to examine social and economic factors that have a major impact on health, well-being, and quality of life. The goal in studying SDOH is to improve health and reduce health disparities. The CDC gives the following examples of SDOH:

- Safe housing, transportation, and neighborhoods.
- Racism, discrimination, and violence.
- Education, job opportunities, and income.
- Access to nutritious foods and physical activity opportunities.
- Polluted air and water.
- Language and literacy skills.

For me, SDOH is far from just an academic term. It's quite personal. I spent my childhood living below the federal poverty line. There were times when we didn't have enough food because my mom, a single mother living in Atlanta, did not make a living wage. Occasionally we even needed public assistance to get by, no matter how hard she worked. Once she and another struggling single mom joined forces to share rent and food stamps, but even after combining resources there still wasn't enough to make it. I can remember one day, on the last day of the month, we had only enough food left to make chili, but bugs had invaded my mother's spices. Mom told me to fish the bugs out. The bug-infested chili was all we had to eat. I couldn't handle the bugs and went hungry. My mother kept a spotless home, but our apartment building was infested with roaches. No matter how often it was sprayed, the pests always came back. When I was ten, my father sent me some money as a gift. He had meant for me to buy something for myself, but instead, I spent that gift money on a new pesticide I'd seen on TV, a foam that was supposed to keep the pests out by sealing up the cracks in the walls. I meticulously filled up every crack in our kitchen. It didn't work. I look back sadly at this vision of a little girl on her hands and knees under the cabinets, trying to get rid of roaches. To this day, I have an acute aversion to the vermin that haunted me as a child.

We tried our best to keep clean, but it cost ten dollars to wash our clothes, so my mom could only afford to go to the laundromat once a month. And without a car it was an ordeal for us just to get there. I faced an even more painful ordeal in elementary school, where I was teased for my dirty clothing.

We didn't have health insurance. I got the shots required to start school and that was it for my medical care. Without the usual childhood preventative care, I ended up catching mumps (a totally vaccine-preventable illness) in college and being quarantined for two weeks. Only once did I see a doctor as a child. I was nine and having severe headaches. My mother saved up the fifty dollars required for a doctor visit. After a quick examination, the doctor pronounced that I was fine. My mom was upset: "I spent all that money to take you to see this doctor and there's nothing wrong with you." Later, I found out that there was indeed something wrong—I had migraines. I diagnosed myself in medical school once I understood that the majority of headaches in women are migraines. That was my first experience of being dismissed by a doctor—at nine years old!

As you can see, I grew up with many of those social determinants of health: lack of transportation, no insurance, not enough food to eat, and unsafe housing. Yes, social determinants of health are a real thing, particularly food insecurity—not having money to pay for food and not having access to healthy food. Four decades later, life for the socially vulnerable hasn't changed much. Their health, or lack of it, is largely determined by social and environmental factors, as was mine.

A Closer Look at Social Determinants of Health

In nineteenth-century Germany, pathologist Rudolf Virchow was sent by the Prussian government to investigate a typhus outbreak in Upper Silesia. Virchow's groundbreaking report identified poverty and social inequity as the principal causes and placed blame on the government's neglect of individuals living in poverty. He prescribed outlawing the feudal system that deprived the underclass of healthy living conditions. The government was displeased with his findings and sent him to war eight days later.

Virchow is revered as an early proponent of social medicine. His report was an early argument that health and well-being are based on factors aside from medical care alone. Virchow saw that where and how people lived was critically important to their health. That people's health depends on economic stability, educational access and quality, neighborhood and built environment, health-care access and quality, social and community context, and racism. These factors are now described as SDOH.

Economic stability varies with race, ethnicity, language, and geographic location. The lower their socioeconomic status, the more barriers people face to positive health-care outcomes. Economic stress can devastate both one's mental and physical health. In the progression of SDOH, economic instability is known as an "upstream determinant," likely to be the source of other social determinants downstream. Economic stability is also directly tied to race. For example, in the United States, Black and Hispanic families have a median wealth that is about one-tenth of White families, regardless of education, marital status, age, or income.

Without healthy finances, educational access and quality will likely suffer. Without a good education, a person is less likely to improve their socioeconomic status. They will struggle to access good health care, adequate housing, and the ability to make healthy life choices. Research has determined that improvements in education, even more than medical care, would have saved eight times more lives across a ten-year span. That's a great argument for investing in education.

Without money or a good education, people may be forced to live in cheaper, unsafe areas. Impoverished racial and ethnic minorities often find themselves trapped in unhealthy urban neighborhoods. In addition to increased violence, residents suffer from unclean water and air. Witness the lead-poisoning crisis in the Flint, Michigan, water system. A 2014 study analyzed nitrogen dioxide concentrations in the air across the United States. Exposure to high levels of NO_2, a byproduct of combustion that causes irritation to the eyes, nose, throat, and lungs when inhaled, increases the chances for hospital stays, asthma, and even cancer. The study found 38 percent higher exposure in non-Whites compared to Whites, due to the proximity of non-White neighborhoods to congested, polluted roads. The research extrapolated that if non-White exposure could be reduced to equal White exposure, seven thousand deaths a year from heart disease could be avoided.

In both urban and rural areas, individuals living in poverty may be unable to afford transportation to medical care. Millions of Americans face these transportation barriers. Urban neighborhood dwellers share barriers to health care with those in impoverished rural areas: Rural dwellers may also have limited access to quality education, food, and health care. Travel for medical care is a time and economic barrier for many rural inhabitants, leading to fewer doctor visits. Add to this our severe physician shortages in rural communities and we find rural underprivileged individuals joining their urban counterparts in the ranks of the medically deprived.

For both urban and rural populations, insurance affordability remains a barrier to health-care access in this country. Those without insurance often don't have a primary care provider. Even with the Affordable Care Act, high deductibles and copays can keep patients from seeking diagnosis and treatment. Preventative care becomes a luxury when it should be a necessity. Fear of out-of-pocket medical costs forces individuals to delay or forgo doctor visits, dental cleanings, medications, and mental health treatment.

Social and community context is another SDOH that is often ignored. These are the connections one has to their community and the people around them. When faced with challenges outside their control, such as an unsafe neighborhood, economic instability, or racial discrimination, a person's positive relationships with family and community can help to reduce the negative impact of these stressors. Lacking such supportive relationships, as in the case of a child whose parents are in jail or a senior who has outlived their family, can contribute to negative health outcomes.

The last SDOH I want to mention is racism, which as a social determinant lives far upstream. From racism flow inequities in housing, income, and education. Racism has such an overarching negative effect on all SDOH that some experts do not classify it as a social determinant at all, but rather as a root cause of SDOH. Either way, racism's effects on health outcomes are clear. As stated by the American Public Health Association following George Floyd's death: "Racism attacks people's physical and mental health. And racism is an ongoing public health crisis that needs our attention now!"

How Poverty Affects Patients

Every week I see patients facing the same issues I had as a child. Two of my patients live in rent-controlled but rodent-infested apartments, as I did. Both want to move because the pests create so much anxiety for them. They asked me to write letters to their landlords in support of their requests to break their leases. I stated my medical opinion that the pests are a danger to my patients' health, but my letter doesn't really matter. They can't move out of the substandard apartments. There is no other housing that they could afford.

Another patient hasn't seen me in person for over a year. I really need to check her vitals often to make sure her congestive heart failure isn't causing fluid overload. The reason she hasn't come to see me is very simple: She doesn't have a ride. Even if she could afford an Uber, she has no smartphone or internet access.

Many people just don't have the money for proper medical care. Some experts propose technology solutions, such as telehealth, to level the playing field. That's a great idea in theory, but for a telehealth visit you need a smartphone or internet access. Online tools and resources could help people manage their heath, but again, you need a smartphone or internet access. That all costs money. In fact, I have patients who don't even have enough money for the copay on their medication. When they run out, they have to wait until the next paycheck or benefit payment.

If you think poverty is an issue for just a few people in America, you are mistaken. According to a report by the National Women's Law Center based on U.S. Census data, in 2019, nearly one in nine women (13.9 million) lived in poverty. Elderly women, women of color, women with disabilities, and families headed by unmarried mothers all faced even higher rates of poverty. More than two in five (46 percent) of those women lived in extreme poverty, defined as income at or below 50 percent of the federal poverty level.

The National Women's Law Center research found that women are 35 percent more likely to live in poverty than men. Women in all racial and ethnic groups were more likely than white, non-Hispanic men to be in poverty. About one in twelve (8 percent) of White women lived in poverty, compared to 6 percent of White men. Poverty rates were particularly high for specific groups of women: 18 percent of Black women, 18 percent of Native American women, and 15 percent of Latinx women. As you recall, these are the groups we have determined likely to feel dismissed because of cultural bias.

And here's something even more alarming—these numbers are all pre-COVID. According to the U.S. Census Bureau, "The official poverty rate in 2020 was 11.4 percent, up one percentage point from 2019. This was the first increase in poverty in years, after five consecutive annual declines. In 2020, there were 37.2 million people in poverty, approximately 3.3 million more than in 2019." Those numbers are expected to get much worse as COVID tears through our vulnerable populations.

The fact is that MANY Americans struggle daily with unemployment, poverty, housing instability, and food insecurity. The pandemic has only amplified economic instability, increasing the risks of poor health outcomes for many already-vulnerable individuals and families. Without the proper resources or support, millions of Americans are unable to afford healthy lifestyle choices or access good medical care. This situation is not new. Poverty due to social inequities has affected the health of people throughout history, as we saw in Virchow's nineteenth-century feudal Prussia. Our society has its own feudal stratifications caused by social determinants of health. Those will not go away without some drastic changes to our world.

The High Cost We All Pay

I have talked about how I was personally affected by SDOH, as well as their effect on my patients. There is also a high cost to society as a whole. By "cost" I am not only talking about people dying unnecessarily, which should affect all of us as human beings. I am talking about money. Our annual national health expenditures have soared to over three trillion dollars. If we continue the current trajectory of spending, the cost will be six trillion dollars by 2028, or 20 percent of our GDP. We are mortgaging our future and the future of our children without even adequately meeting our current needs.

According to 2017 numbers from the Agency for Healthcare Research and Quality (AHRQ), 1 percent of the United States population accounted for 22 percent of our health-care spending. Five percent accounted for more than 50 percent of health-care expenditures. Those are astounding figures. Decision-makers in the health-care system have tried to identify the high utilizers and intervene to reduce costs. They apply a risk stratification formula, assigning a risk score to each patient. Patients with higher risk scores are more likely to accumulate costs for medical care.

Developed in 2002 at the University of California at San Diego, the most common risk-calculation method for Medicaid populations is the Chronic Illness and Disability Payment System (CDPS) combined with prescription costs. This method combines medical and psychiatric risk in one score. Although widely used, the CDPS + Rx formula has shown little improvement from "hot spotting," which targeted the sickest, highest utilizers in health plans. Recent research points to SDOHs as key drivers of health outcomes and health-care spending. One new SDOH-based risk model would separately address each of a patient's risks from medical diagnoses, psychiatric diagnoses, and social determinants of health. This would allow for segmenting risk and taking focused actions based on those risks.

I feel strongly that we need to factor in the bias that may cause vulnerable patients to utilize the health-care system in more expensive ways. Is our biased treatment of Black patients sending them to more expensive emergency rooms and urgent care centers? Is the lack of unbiased specialists willing to go into women's health or senior health costing us more and putting additional financial burdens on our economy?

With the recent increased stress on our health-care system, it is even more critical that we find a formula to accurately calculate risk. We know that doctors and nurses are feeling burned-out. Many plan to leave health care. We will not have enough medical providers to take care of a growing sick and aging population. We must address the core social problems that are the root causes of health disparities. We must base our work on SDOH. We must acknowledge that our country's health crisis is socially determined.

CHAPTER 13

Science as an Invasive Health-Care Influence

THE ECONOMIC AND SOCIAL CHALLENGES resulting in Social Determinants of Health (SDOH) are further complicated by forces that we do not usually associate with health equity. I have created an acronym for them: Invasive Health-Care Influences in America (IHIA). Yes, another acronym, but I believe the idea of invasive influences may be useful to characterize how these forces have penetrated our health-care system. I'm thinking of the Tree of Heaven analogy I used earlier in the discussion of bias. As a reminder, the Tree of Heaven is highly invasive and does a great deal of harm by killing other species. Just like bias. This tree is the bane of many a gardener's life. We not-so-jokingly call it the Tree of Hell. Yet, I was unaware until lately that the Tree of Heaven also does good things, like regenerating soil by absorbing contaminants, adding green to urban landscapes that can't support other trees, serving as an ozone bioindicator, and hosting silkworms in places where birds are less likely to prey on caterpillars. In some ways the Tree of Hell is the Tree of Heaven.

The influences that I call "invasive" are institutions like social and traditional media, technology, research, product development, religion, educational systems. They are ubiquitous in health care and have both good and bad effects on health equity. Among the IHIAs, science has been on my mind over the last few years, specifically the bias *against* science that is interfering with the relationship between health-care providers and patients.

Bias against science bewilders me. Since I was young girl, I have *loved* science. It's one of the reasons I became an engineer and then a doctor. A highly curious person, I love solving problems. I am fascinated by the scientific method. I can't imagine a world without the medical breakthroughs from science: anesthesia, artificial insulin, gene therapy, medical imaging, organ transplants, and immunotherapy, to name just a few.

I'm familiar with anti-science bias from some of my patients, as with their resistance to the flu vaccine. I have noticed that one subgroup of my patient population has a very low flu-shot adoption rate (approximately 40 percent) and they are predominantly African American. Many of these patients willingly accept other vaccines like tetanus, pneumonia, and even the vaccination to prevent shingles. But when it comes to the flu shot, they say, "Oh no, I don't do flu shots." I have yet to understand the reasoning behind this singular vaccine refusal. Many of these patients have health conditions that make them just as vulnerable to influenza as they are to COVID. None of my arguments or scientific evidence have changed their resolve. Here I am a Black woman doctor explaining to other Black women that the flu shot is safe, yet they still decline the vaccine, against my medical advice. I explain that they face the highest risk of ending up in the ICU of any racial group, and they still decline the vaccine. They respect me and know that I care deeply for them as patients and people, but that doesn't sway them at all.

Frankly, I am perplexed. To me, vaccination against the flu, COVID, and other diseases is a no-brainer. Globally, an estimated 37 million lives were saved between 2000 and 2019 because of vaccinations. Of course, COVID has taken a huge physical and emotional toll on every health provider I know. I was elated when the vaccines finally came out, but then deeply disheartened when so many people rejected what I considered a miracle. My spirits were lifted when I saw that the majority of patients in our practice did accept the COVID vaccine, much higher than the national average. I give credit to my team, who worked very hard to address concerns one-on-one, and really *listened* to what people were worried about. I am proud to be part of the medical and scientific community that has developed this miraculous vaccine. It makes me sad when patients decline vaccines that I know will protect them against preventable illnesses, but I understand that the high vaccine denial rate is an example of how deep medical mistrust runs in our community.

The Increase in "Know-It-All" Bias

Resistance to vaccines and other medical treatment is one type of anti-science bias that I witness as a doctor. Another bias that I have seen growing in recent years is what I call "know-it-all" bias. A patient gets "medical" information from friends or Dr. Google that is not evidence-based, but they accept it as fact. This is illustrated in a cartoon of a man sitting at his computer as his wife walks by. The caption: "Honey, come look! I found some information all the world's top scientists and doctors missed!"

I do believe strongly in shared decision-making between health-care providers and their patients. Your body is your body. My job is to diagnose and treat it based on accepted and proven standards of medicine. Your job is to listen to my recommendations and work with me on choosing a solution that will produce the best outcomes. We consider not just physical outcomes but also how a treatment will affect you mentally and spiritually.

We do appreciate a patient who comes prepared and knowledgeable to a doctor visit. But that is very different than a patient who tells me what their diagnosis is, based on misinformation, before I even have a chance to examine them. Being prepared is great. But I don't appreciate being told that I am recommending a procedure just to make more money. Being knowledgeable is not telling me that their great-grandma used vinegar to cure a disease, so that's good enough for them. All these things have happened to me and other medical providers.

Medically literate patients are easier to work with, because they can weigh the options and make informed, objective choices. They understand that every treatment has risk factors, and diagnosis is not always foolproof. You could take an aspirin and have a reaction to it, but the vast odds are that you will not. If you have seen the endless list of possible side effects in TV drug commercials, you know that you always need to weigh benefits with risk. That list of possible side effects, by the way, is the result of intensive clinical drug trials and is required by law. I also firmly believe that patients should have questions for me from knowing their own bodies. Andrew Folts, a blogger, YouTuber, and creative colleague of Kathy's, articulates this in "What Good Is Science if We Can't Question the System Behind It?" which I have included here with his permission.

> In elementary school, the first thing I ever learned about science was the scientific method: "Observe, Hypothesize, Test, Analyze, Report." I loved conducting self-experiments, and when I started going bald in college, I spent months researching studies, but after a year of taking a hair-loss medication my doctor assured me was "safe," my libido was totally gone.
>
> From there I started noticing other problems: deodorant rashes, antihistamine drowsiness, nasal spray nosebleeds, and digestive chaos from "scientifically verified" diets, each of which contradicted the others. Finally, following a flu shot in 2019, I developed chronic, body-wide joint inflammation that has yet to resolve.

It felt like the "science" I loved as a kid had betrayed me at every turn, and worse, I didn't even know why.

Yesterday Joe Rogan released an interview with Dr. Robert Malone (who helped develop mNRA), and it clarified a point I've been conflicted on for years, which is that... [d]enying "science" and raising questions about the system behind it are not the same thing. It's convenient to believe that health is a monolith—that one treatment is "safe" and "effective" for everyone, but the human body is more complicated than that, and although science is unassailable, people are not.

By pretending financial bias does not exist, by discounting individual experience, and by de-platforming anyone who challenges the default narrative, we're turning reality into a court case with no prosecution. Obviously it's foolish to believe every word spilled into a podcast mic, but people have a right to speak, and one day our lives might depend on whether we listen. *What good is science in a bad system? Truth only survives when we question both sides.*

As a doctor, I appreciate Andrew's thoughtful views from a patient perspective. I do wonder if his sensitivity to various products and the flu shot has an underlying cause that has not yet been detected. But in Andrew's case I don't think that, by choosing to ignore conventional medical wisdom, he is taking risks to his health. He can select deodorants without the chemicals that he is sensitive to. Nasal sprays are generally just for discomfort, so he is fine in avoiding them. It is important to know your personal reaction to certain foods, and one should not blindly follow diets. Andrew is a young, athletic man, not an older person who could die from flu complications. I'm okay with his refusing the flu shot if it causes him harm. In fact, I think his proactivity and self-awareness are good for his health. He is right that we all react differently to medications. If I have a patient who complains of a reaction to a medication, I immediately pull them off it. I reintroduce the medication later, and if the reaction reoccurs, I have evidence that the medication is to blame for that patient's reaction. That's the scientific method.

Andrew practices health literacy and engages in healthy, educated skepticism. I love patients like him. Let me contrast him with the patients who attacked health-care providers like Kathryn Ivey, a critical care nurse during the COVID crisis. In a poignant essay, she describes what it is like for her and her colleagues working day in and day out to save the lives of (often) unvaccinated patients during COVID. I read this essay with tears in my eyes and a great appreciation for these tireless frontline health-care workers. Kathryn has been active in the media, including a thread on Twitter chronicling her first year as a nurse during the pandemic.

While many thanked her, others did not: "As the comments (that I tried not to read) rolled in, I learned that I'm a fake, crisis actor. I'm getting paid to make COVID look worse than it is. I'm getting paid when my patients die." She was told to give them ivermectin and that ventilators kill patients. She even received comments that nurses and doctors are murderers. "I wish I could say that these comments had no effect on me, but many of them, especially the ones accusing me and my colleagues of killing our patients, hit like a punch in the gut."

Kathryn has received death threats and refuses to publicly identify where she works because of fear for herself and her colleagues. She mentions a TikTok video where a man caught on a security camera threatens the nurses and doctors who he believes killed his friend with treatment, stating he has a gun at home and has been studying the nurses' routines. "My in-person experiences with individuals who would threaten nurses physically or sue a hospital to force them to administer ivermectin or hydroxychloroquine, have been small but not zero. Each has left me angry and unsettled, at a total loss to understand how anyone could think that we wouldn't end this misery in a heartbeat if we could," she concludes.

How Did We Get Here

There is a huge difference between healthy skepticism with shared decision-making versus dismissal of medical treatment and threats against providers. How did we reach a place in America where we can be so fearful, angry, and resentful about science and, specifically, medical science? This attitude has always existed in parts of our society and throughout the world and has often been influenced by politics and religion. Think of classic literature like *Frankenstein* and *Dr. Jekyll and Mr. Hyde*, which portrayed a mad scientist whose thirst for knowledge drives him beyond the societal view of what is right or wrong.

Academics have studied the anti-science phenomenon in history, politics, philosophy, psychology, and ethics. Andrew Jewett is associate professor of history at Harvard University and author of *Science Under Fire: Challenges to Scientific Authority in Modern America*. Jewett says skepticism about science goes back to the 1920s, when cultural critics were alarmed about the influence of science on social changes. These critics believed that science violated conventional morality and encouraged teaching sex education in biology classes. They included mandatory vaccination programs in their list of science's invasions of public morals.

"To fully explain today's distrust of science, we must account for the longstanding fear that it authorizes false and damaging understandings of who we are and how we behave," he writes. He argues that it is not just conservatives who question scientific authority in America. Instead, he says alarm about application of biological research crosses party lines in areas like genetic engineering and biotechnology. People tend to pick and choose among scientific theories and applications, based on preexisting commitments.

Robert Crease, a philosophy professor at Stony Brook University, responded to the question "What is the difference between science denial, anti-science, pseudoscience, and skepticism?" in Quora, a social question-and-answer website. His answer was later showcased in *Fortune* magazine. He explains that science denial is accepting science for most things but denying it for things you don't like. He gives the example of being told by a doctor that you have a disease that requires a costly and painful cure. "If I refuse to take the cure from my doctor whom I've relied on for years and tell him or her that 'I don't have that disease!' or 'That's the wrong cure!' that's science denial. There's no evidence, and I am not qualified to make the judgment."

In comparison to science denial, anti-science is doubting the advice of all doctors because they can't be trusted. Someone who is anti-science rejects science and scientific method, the foundation of evidence-based medicine. "Those engaged in anti-science don't pretend to think scientifically or even want to. Anti-science is mainly an attitude, a personal response. You therefore can't respond to it by throwing more science at me." Pseudoscience and skepticism are both different than science denial and anti-science. Pseudoscience passes off false, unreliable, or unproven claims as scientific. The pseudoscientist promotes a cure for their own benefit, with no proof behind it. Skepticism involves doubting a specific finding for specific reasons. For example, you might not take a doctor's advice, based on your own investigations into other evidence-based treatments. Denying science and being skeptical can look similar. The difference, according to Crease, is that science denial undermines institutions like medicine and is motivated by the pursuit of economic, religious, political, or other agendas.

That statement did not surprise me and is supported by research. The science denial used to deny the existence of the pandemic and refuse its restrictions was more associated with political affiliation than with factors directly connected to the disease, such as age. A 10 percent increase in Fox News viewership led to a reduction in people staying at home during the height of the pandemic. Republican-led states had lower case counts and deaths from COVID-19 early on in the pandemic, but higher rates from June through December 2020, adjusting for factors like age, race, poverty, and obesity.

There is questioning of science in America, but the majority of Americans do have confidence in science. In Gallup Polls' annual Confidence in Institutions survey, 64 percent of respondents said they had "a great deal" or "quite a lot" of confidence in science, which puts science among the highest of seventeen institutions, behind small business and the military. But look at the difference among political partisans: Republicans are much less likely to have confidence in science; Democrats today have more confidence. The current survey shows a thirty-four-point difference in science-confidence levels between the two parties, the largest gap since the question was first asked in 1975, and is among the largest Gallup has ever measured for any institution.

Making Americans Believe in Science

Americans are endangering their health by being anti-science, denying science, or using treatments without supporting evidence. We must recognize the different kinds of science bias and their historical contexts in order to target appropriate strategies against them.

First, we need to depoliticize science. I have no clue how to do that except by being active voters and change agents who watch for politicians from both parties who push a get-elected election agenda instead of a socially beneficial agenda. I also think that the scientific community needs to get much more vocal when they see politics interfering with science, particularly in institutions that most Americans trust like the CDC and FDA.

Second, we need to realize that for some groups, science bias is directly connected to racism. The histories of Black Americans and Native Americans provide strong reasons why members of those groups would be science averse. We need to get many more minorities into science roles, especially in medicine, and push minority scientists into leadership positions. They can be the change agents who can work directly with their communities to overcome barriers to science.

Third, we need to make science people-friendly, instead of hiding it in laboratories and couching it in complex language. People are naturally curious about their world, so accessible science would be a huge help in alleviating fear and distrust. One strategy might be to link it to America's love of celebrities. For example, acceptance of mental health issues has taken a big leap forward in the last decade as public figures have started talking candidly about their struggles. And maybe we can marshal the support of Captain America, Spider-Man, Hulk, and Iron Man, who are all scientists in the Marvel universe.

Fourth, we need to make sure science education begins at the earliest age, when children are sponges for learning. We can teach the scientific method and experimentation to children. Unfortunately, the early-education programs that do this now work through elite institutions like museums, which are financially and geographically inaccessible to many people. But models in other early-education areas, like reading, have produced great results through private-public participation. Dolly Parton's Imagination Library comes to mind. Maybe we need Dolly to take on science as her next project.

Fifth, we all need to respond to skepticism in constructive ways. For health-care providers, this means not dismissing our patients because we are weary or running to the next appointment. It means not taking their questions as an affront to our training and expertise. For patients, it means not making assumptions about how your doctor will react or treating them in a disrespectful manner. It means being as prepared as they are with evidence-based research so you can work with them on treatment decisions. For both, embracing skepticism in healthy ways means trying to check your biases at the door.

Since the Renaissance, science has "invaded" health care. We have moved away from spells and incantations and toward the scientific method to back up our medical treatments. That's a good thing, a welcome invasion. Like that pesky Tree of Heaven, science has grown by facing the realities of its physical conditions, finding ways of survival through experimentation and persistence.

CHAPTER 14

Technology as an Invasive Health-Care Influence

D R. LEONARD "BONES" MCCOY ON *Star Trek* was a beloved TV doctor. He kept the crew of the USS *Enterprise* fit to "boldly go where no man has gone before." His sick bay was stocked with magical space-age medical technology. But, as Bones put it when admonishing First Officer Spock, "I'm not a magician, Spock, just an old country doctor."

Speaking from the future in science fiction, Bones's statement cleverly alludes to some real issues with today's developing medical technology. First, no matter how good the technology, health-care providers are not magicians. Technology can provide unprecedented access to health care and lower costs, but technology will not cure the health inequities faced by so many. In fact, some believe that it will widen the gap between the haves and the have-nots. Second, patients still want their "old country doctor," a trustworthy human being. Health care built exclusively on technology, without the patient-physician connection, will inevitably fall short. We already hear patients complain about doctors more focused on their computers than on the person on the examining table.

The medical future in *Star Trek* of the 1960s promised a world where treatment and diagnosis are instant and accurate. Bones had a medical "tricorder," a handheld scanner that instantly checked vital organ functions and detected the presence of disease. Now we're trying to make that come true: A technology race is currently underway sixty years later to bring this diagnostic device to consumers for home use. To spur innovation, the Qualcomm Tricorder X Prize promised $10 million to the first team to build a medical tricorder that could diagnose fifteen medical conditions ranging from sleep apnea to colon cancer. No team's invention met all the winning criteria, but they did make progress toward bringing this technology to its huge potential market.

Who knows what the future will bring for self-diagnostic technology? The inventors will need to address concerns from both doctors and regulators about the risks of self-diagnosis. Bones, the doctor, used the tricorder to diagnose *Enterprise* crew members. They never used it on themselves. But Americans are clamoring for technology that would empower them to control their own health. We're crazy for Fitbits, phone health apps, home monitors for blood pressure, blood glucose, and heart rate. We may not have *Star Trek* tricorders yet, but we're getting there. We will have to deal with the ethical and professional issues of self-diagnosis once we get there.

The initial price tag for portable diagnostic scanners will be high. Remember that the first cell phone was $3,995 in 1984, when it was first released. That's the equivalent of $9,952 in 2020 dollars. Today the average price of a smartphone is $208. When they finally hit the market, portable body-scanners may be accessible only to the rich, but the price for the average person will likely come down over time. When access to these technologies becomes open to all, I think it may help alleviate some effects of the racial and cultural bias that now cause unequal access to health care.

Empowering Patients with Technology

Though the *Star Trek* tricorder is still in the future, we do have two kinds of technology that put patients in the driver's seat: products and services that monitor and screen for health risks, conditions, and diseases; and communication technologies that put patients in touch with their health-care providers.

Let's look at the first category. The self-diagnostic-products market is predicted to reach almost $9 billion globally by 2027, and that's probably a low-ball estimate. Currently we have self-testing for pregnancy, blood sugar, colon cancer, infectious diseases like hepatitis, HIV, and COVID as well as genetic tests that check for higher risk for certain diseases. Some of these tests give you immediate results, while others need to be sent to a lab. Many are affordable and easily purchased at pharmacies or online.

At-home monitoring and wearables will also improve the patient's access to their health information, particularly when costs come down. A company my practice works with has made in-home blood pressure monitoring affordable and easy with a Bluetooth-enabled blood pressure cuff. This doesn't require our patients to have home Wi-Fi, which many cannot afford. It is simple to use, which helps our patients who are older or have disabilities. Every time they check their blood pressure, the cuff automatically transmits their numbers to our office. It has been a big help to our office by keeping our eyes on vulnerable patients when we can't see them in person.

Technology also now allows people to get a more comprehensive picture of their health with innovations like genomics, cancer blood tests, MRIs, and sleep analysis. With this information, individuals can take a proactive and personalized approach to their own health. A full-body MRI scan can detect problems like brain tumors, spinal deterioration, and heart disease before the onset of symptoms. New blood tests can screen for more than fifty kinds of cancer. These technologies are still very expensive, so now they are just being used as a benefit for some corporate executives or purchased by wealthy individuals. They are not yet available to the average person, and certainly not to the disadvantaged.

Insurance companies do not always cover the new screening technologies unless a patient is showing symptoms of a disorder, even if they have a family history of a disease. This is a shame, since these scans can give doctors and patients so much information. Scanning technology will get cheaper as it gets older, but in the meantime, we are missing many opportunities for early diagnosis, which could help avoid frustration and heartbreak. One of my patients, Evelyn, developed type one diabetes in her late fifties. This is unusual, since type 1 diabetes normally begins in childhood. An adult can develop this disease if they have pancreatic cancer. My patient's specialist wanted her to get a CAT scan of her abdomen to rule this out. At that point, she had no pain, so the insurance company denied coverage, and she could not afford to pay several thousand dollars for the scan. Two months later when Evelyn developed pain, insurance allowed the scan, but by then she was diagnosed with stage four pancreatic cancer. She died. Would an earlier CAT scan have saved her life? I don't know, but I believe it would have given her more of a chance.

Because of stories like Evelyn's, I have become an advocate for self-pay options. Diagnostic imaging packages include screens to check for blockages in your arteries, aortic aneurisms, and an echocardiogram to check for heart failure or anatomical anomalies that may not cause symptoms until later in life. The service was very expensive at first, but prices are coming down so more people can afford it. These scans are particularly valuable for middle-aged people who want to assess their future health risks. I also encourage my patients to open health saving accounts (HSAs) to pay for services that insurance will not authorize. The HSA allows you to put pre-tax dollars aside for future out-of-pocket health-care expenses and can be used to meet your insurance deductible. For some accounts, unused funds can roll over to the next year and eventually become a retirement instrument.

Now let's look at technologies that help patients communicate with health-care providers. Patient portals and telemedicine have had the widest adoption by health-care systems. Patient portals allow patients to schedule appointments, message their health-care team, review their records, and see lab reports. They allow for sharing of medical charts with multiple providers. In 2020, nearly 40 percent of Americans accessed a patient portal, most often to view test results. The patients who chose not to use the portal said their main reason was that they preferred to speak to a health-care provider directly.

Surveys show that rural residents and individuals with less education and lower household incomes were less likely to access their available patient portals. The groups less likely to be offered the use of a patient portal were men, middle-aged adults, racial or ethnic minorities, those with less education and lower household incomes, those who do not use the internet, and those living in rural areas.

Surveys have shown that while minority patients were significantly less likely to enroll in portals, once enrolled, they used portals in the same ways as other groups. The oldest patients were less likely to enroll, citing privacy and security concerns and either lack of access to or the inability to use technology as their most common barriers. Younger patients were more likely to enroll, but less likely to use the portal to solicit provider advice or request medication. Male patients were less likely than women to use the portal to solicit provider advice.

If we want to increase the use of patient portals by groups who experience racial and cultural bias, we need to direct training and communication at their specific needs. The same holds true for telemedicine. I believe that telemedicine offers great advantages to patients. Drive times to my office can be long, and many of my patients are already short of time from their jobs, family, and caregiver responsibilities. It seemed like a no-brainer to me that they would love video appointments, where they wouldn't need to take off work, drive, or arrange babysitting. I was an early adopter of telemedicine, but my patients were not. I think they were afraid that we could not accurately or reliably diagnose them by video. They would say things like, "I need her to see me," or "I need you to see what's going on." They did not understand that telemedicine still works—we still have patients get blood work, X-rays, and other diagnostic tests in person.

We don't do the hands-on physical exam, but with the visual input, tests, and medical history, telemedicine is still reliable for many cases. In cases where we can't diagnose and treat without a physical exam, we see the patient in person.

The COVID lockdown made telemedicine essential, so we were glad to have our system already in place. Our telemedicine system was up and running when our offices needed to close. Now our patients are used to the technology and comfortable with it, but they still prefer in-person appointments. I'm not surprised by that—one survey found that while 82 percent of people reported satisfaction with telemedicine experiences, 64 percent would have preferred to see their nurse or doctor in person.

Improving the Provider Experience

Electronic medical record technology (EMR) has enhanced the efficiency of medical offices by automating scheduling, creating referrals, electronically filling prescriptions, and centralizing access to medical records and data. We can now see test results in one place and have multiple people view a chart at the same time. When I first started medicine, the joke was that there was always at least one person walking around our facility looking for a patient chart. One doctor might have the chart on their desk because they're still working on their notes, or the nurse might have pulled the chart because they had to fax over a prescription refill for the patient. On rare occasions, the chart might even have been misfiled, which was a big deal since we had to figure out how to make a new one. And once the chart was found, we still had to read the doctors' terrible handwriting. EMR changed all that.

These efficiencies are great, but I particularly appreciate EMRs for quality improvements in patient safety and clinical outcomes. EMRs incorporate decision-support algorithms that help identify and prevent medical errors, such as medication errors, by checking for drug allergies, potential drug interactions, and dosing. The systems also facilitate communication among doctors, nurses, and pharmacists to resolve analog errors like bad handwriting.

Many patients who have experienced racial and cultural bias also have multiple medical conditions that require more monitoring and testing than other patients. EMRs capture, record, and analyze the clinical information needed to treat these patients. These patients often see multiple specialists, and EMRs improve care coordination, reducing errors and redundant tests by allowing medical-record sharing.

EMRs allow doctors to take an overall look at their patient population as well as to see patterns in individual patient data. This means I can look at common problems among my patients and then develop strategies and programs for better outcomes. For example, if I notice that certain groups of my patients are experiencing more high blood pressure, I can analyze that data by any variables I choose. Is that trend related to race? Type of job? Marital status? Diagnosis of anxiety or depression? This ease of data analysis helps my team provide care targeted to my patients' needs.

Finally, EMRs allow doctors to provide more personal care because all the patient's information is at our fingertips. The provider-patient relationship is less personal these days. We have less time during appointments and are seeing people less frequently than we should. With all their information immediately available, we providers can prepare ourselves to address the whole person. For example, our EMR has a secure area where we can put in little notes about the patient, such as a recent loss, what name they preferred to be called by, or even if they are planning to climb Mount Kilimanjaro. When we see that patient, we can look them in the eye and connect human to human.

As with any technology, EMRs have their downsides. Initially, some patients thought it was cool to have a computer in the examining room, where we could automatically send a prescription to the pharmacy. In fact, I had one patient who complained because a doctor didn't bring the computer into the room with her. She wanted to see all the results of her recent X-rays and labs. But many patients do not like the loss of eye contact. Patients want their doctors to be looking at them, not entering data into a computer. Here are some comments we received on our Pulse Survey:

> Looking at numbers and not listening to what I am saying.

> He doesn't even look at me, just the screen.

> Has his face in the computer and never looks at me.

> The current practice of using computer records during appointments: This makes me as a patient feel irrelevant to the interaction. That's not really the provider's fault, but I think the provider can make an effort to speak directly with the patient more of the time.

That makes perfect sense to me. Earlier, we talked about the need to practice compassion, empathy, and respect for all patients, but particularly for those who have been routinely dismissed by the health-care system. What is more dismissive than looking at a computer when there is a human being sitting next to you? Any of us who have tried to communicate with our teenagers or spouses whose eyes never leave their phones know how it feels to be invisible. Why should our patients have to feel like that?

In my patient encounters I focus on eye contact and then let the patient know when I am about to input some notes. Then I bring my focus back to the patient. My computer is always to the side, while my body and face are turned to the patient. This is difficult for some doctors. They haven't been trained as data entry clerks. In fact, many doctors don't type well or are not adept with computers. They don't learn typing or computer usage in medical school, yet we're now responsible for typing and capturing all this data. If the doctor is struggling with the technology, that's a further distraction from the patient. Can you imagine an attorney in a courtroom having to type everything they're saying while giving their arguments?

One solution is to employ a medical scribe who comes to the examining room with you and records data in real time. This lets the provider concentrate on the patient and not use valuable time typing. Medical scribes are like court reporters. But scribes cost money, and this is just another expense for already-stretched primary care practices. Medical scribes are not billable to insurance, nor are doctors compensated for the time they put in keeping patient records accurate and up to date. Our lives would be much easier if there were an insurance code for medical scribes.

Patient portals have improved life for providers by facilitating communication with patients. But this has also opened a Pandora's box—some patients overuse or misuse the patient portal. Some ask the provider to diagnose and treat via email. Portal communications are more appropriate for following up on an in-person visit with a simple "I'm doing fine," or "I'm not doing fine." The patient can then request another appointment or referral. Doctors cannot diagnose and treat somebody over a portal message. Patients have sent me paragraphs describing symptoms: "I'm writing because, yesterday I woke up and my back was hurting on the left side and now I have pain down my leg. What should I do?" That's a topic for a visit, not a portal request. Chronic offenders repeatedly use the portal for medical questions and then are upset when we tell them they need an appointment. The art and science of doctoring, diagnosis, and treatment can't be accomplished through an email exchange.

Technology has invaded health care, but I think mostly in good ways. It has the potential to solve so many problems of racial and cultural bias as soon as we can get equity in cost to the patient. But if we use technology to dismiss the patient or as a substitute for the patient-provider relationship, not only will we see worse outcomes, but we will lose a bit of what makes us all human. Health providers and patients have a shared responsibility to use technology to encourage compassion, empathy, and respect. Historically vulnerable groups should be represented in technology research and development, and we should aim our technological progress toward improving human lives.

CHAPTER 15

Pharma and Research
as an Invasive
Health-Care Influence

S O FAR, WE'VE EXAMINED HOW attitudes toward science and the onslaught of new technology have affected health care and, specifically, how they are influenced by racial and cultural bias. Bias is also inherent in pharmaceutical companies and university-based research, which have huge roles on our health-care system, raising many questions. Where does funding come from? How are investments made? How are those resources allocated? How are studies designed and conducted? How is research data generated, how is it used and by whom? Who evaluates research? How do papers reach publication? Who is making those decisions? How does industry-academic collaboration work? What are the mechanisms for advancement of science? How is knowledge transferred back and forth among industry, academia, medical practitioners, and the people?

That's a lot of questions, and I would not presume to try to answer them here. That's a different book—a very large book. But I would like to give you a broad overview of why and how pharma and research have become such an Invasive Health-Care Influence in America (IHIA).

How Drugs Are Developed

Americans spend upwards of $348 billion on prescription drugs each year. I'm amazed, though not surprised, that most patients don't know how these drugs get into their medicine cabinets. My "amazed" reaction is because prescription drugs are such a big part of our lives. I'm not surprised, because getting a drug to market is a complicated process that most people don't understand. But you do need to understand that process to see how it is interwoven with racial and cultural bias.

Drugs are developed with the goal of producing good patient outcomes safely. There are essentially five steps: discovery and development, preclinical research, clinical research, FDA review and approval, and FDA safety monitoring once the drug is in the market. Discovery and development often take place in university research labs and hospitals with funding from government entities like the National Institute of Health (NIH). At this stage, researchers are looking for new insights into a disease process and evaluating compounds for treatment. The preclinical research step makes sure the potential drug does not cause serious harm before testing on humans. Then come multiple clinical trials on volunteers, increasing the number of people being tested with each trial. The developer applies for a patent. With successful trials, the drug is submitted for review and approval by the FDA. If approved, the drug goes to market, where it is still monitored by the FDA. The producer holds the patent, sets the price, and earns revenue until the patent expires. Then the drug can be produced generically, with the price set by the generic producers.

Bias can enter the process at many stages. For example, who received funding during discovery and development stage? Were there steps during preclinical research that were influenced by socioeconomic bias? Did the clinical trials include subjects representative of all races, genders, and age groups? How does the producer position the drug in the market? Do marketing campaigns stereotype or ignore some prescribers and consumers? Will doctors be invited to submit patient data back to researchers on the drug's real-world effects on all potential groups of users?

Inclusion in Clinical Trials and Data Analysis

Historically, clinical trials excluded many of the vulnerable groups we have talked about in this book. It wasn't considered important to consider factors like race and gender. Studies were done on White men with the assumption that what worked for them would also work for people of color and women. That's not what happened.

Women experience adverse drug reactions (ADR) nearly twice as often as men. In one study, researchers from the University of California, Berkeley, and the University of Chicago analyzed data from thousands of articles in medical journals. They found a gender difference in appropriate drug doses for eighty-six medications approved by the FDA, which they attributed to pharmacokinetics (PK), the movement of drugs through bodies. Even when women were included in clinical trials, reported data was not separated out by gender. The researchers concluded: "Sex differences in pharmacokinetics strongly predict sex-specific ADRs for women but not men. This sex difference was not explained by sex differences in body weight. The absence of sex-stratified PK information in public records for hundreds of drugs raises the concern that sex differences in PK values are widespread and of clinical significance."

As new treatments are developed for common diseases, the lack of representative inclusion is troubling. Minority populations have been underrepresented in cancer-drug clinical trials for immunotherapy, but we need to know how those drugs work in the unique biology of the host and the tumors in those subpopulations. Researchers have found that Black patients constitute less than 4 percent of the patients enrolled in trials for immune checkpoint inhibitors for the treatment of lung cancer. We physicians want to consider cancer immunotherapy as a treatment option for our minority patients, but knowing those drugs were not developed for our patients makes us concerned about the outcomes.

Unfortunately, as researchers are finally waking up to the need for inclusion in clinical trials, they are running up against resistance to participate from potential Black volunteers who are aware of the history of abuse of minorities in scientific research. Remember Henrietta Lacks and the Tuskegee experiment? Let me take a second to remind you. In the case of Henrietta Lacks, her cervical cancer cells were kept for research at Johns Hopkins without her informed consent or permission.

In the Tuskegee experiment, for forty years African American men were research subjects in a United States government–sanctioned study to observe the natural history of untreated syphilis. The researchers deceived the subjects using placebos, known ineffective methods, and diagnostic procedures disguised as "treatment." The men who had syphilis were never informed of their diagnosis, despite the risk of infecting others. They were never told that the disease could lead to blindness, deafness, brain damage, heart disease, bone deterioration, and death. They were never offered a cure, though a cure was available.

Why would Black people want to participate in medical research when it has allowed these crimes against humanity? We haven't forgotten.

People of color (and I think the general public) are suspicious of "informed consent" forms, whether for a research study or medical procedure. You would never buy a house or car without having time to read the fine print, but informed consent forms are difficult to understand and presented at the last moment. No wonder some people dig in their heels and refuse to sign these forms that would allow treatment or research participation. People are then concerned about what happens to them when they don't consent to participate in a study that their doctor is recommending or involved in. I've had several patients tell me that they felt that their specialist acted differently after they refused to be part of a study. One patient with congestive heart failure was concerned that her doctor might treat her less effectively because she did not want to be part of his research. That is a horrible burden to place on patients.

We need to be very thoughtful about how we recruit people for studies. We may have assumed that money or participation for the greater good of society would be incentives for anyone, including people of color. But those incentives aren't inviting to those who are scared that something bad is going to be done to them or if society hasn't been all that good to them. You don't trust or respect a White-dominated world that has never had your interests in mind.

Researchers met with that resistance and mistrust when trying to recruit African American patients into trials for the COVID vaccine. They finally succeeded in finding volunteers through churches, which are a central part of African American communities. Many volunteers responded well when respected Black leaders and celebrities talked about participating in terms of Black pride.

Different Approaches
for Research and Researchers

Women and people of color in research positions suffer because of bias that affects both their careers and the contributions they can make. We know that from countless studies. Some organizations with explicit policies and overt agendas for reducing bias still perpetuate it in the workplace. The National Institutes of Health have been addressing the need for inclusion in clinical studies for decades. NIH is a major funder of medical research. Yet even in the NIH, funding proposal reviewers and committee chairs are more likely to be men. Women are more likely to have just temporary affiliations or serve on review committees with lower funding and fewer research grants to award, so have less opportunity to influence the nation's research agenda.

We have opportunities to shape data analysis to look more closely at trends in social determinants of health and minority issues. We have the data sets and technology to analyze the data by subgroups. If my electronic medical records system allows me to collect data and cross-analyze by different variables, then researchers in pharmaceutical companies and universities can do the same. This requires an attitude shift in research design. We should routinely plan into research the analysis of results across vulnerable populations. Any product that will eventually be used across the whole population should be developed with awareness of the SDOH that are such a foundational influence in many lives.

Finally, we need more collaboration and knowledge transfer among patients, clinicians, and researchers. The rare-disease advocacy associations have developed an organizational model that unites patients, doctors' organizations, families, and researchers into one community to move their agenda forward. They raise funds, post current research and regulation, showcase doctors who specialize in that disease, and build patient and family forums. We saw this strategy work powerfully during the AIDS epidemic.

This strategy could be helpful to African Americans. Following George Floyd's murder, Dr. Alexandra Power-Hays and Dr. T. McGann shared their views about racism and Sickle Cell Disease (SCD), often considered a Black disease: "Medicine is a mirror for the racial injustice in our society; it is a field riddled with racial disparities in everything from research funding to patient care to life expectancy." They explained that SCD patients' health care and outcomes may be more affected by racism than patients with other diseases, are often marginalized, and are dismissed when seeking medical care.

The authors called on medical leaders to take action: "Although SCD was first described more than a hundred years ago, the development of disease-modifying therapies has stagnated because of inadequate research funding, attributable at least in part to structural racism." They compared SCD to cystic fibrosis, which primary affects White Americans. One third the number of people get cystic fibrosis, but it receives seven to eleven times the research funding per patient. The FDA has approved four medications for SCD and fifteen for cystic fibrosis. The Cystic Fibrosis Foundation is a huge fundraiser and education source. The Sickle Cell Association of America exists but receives much less funding and media attention.

Changing the Leadership Landscape

In 2020, research and development spending in the pharmaceutical and medical technology industry in the United States totaled nearly $96 billion. The largest investment was in biopharmaceuticals at 52 percent, followed by medical technology at 10 percent. Six of the top pharmaceutical companies in the world are headquartered in the United States. In 2019, universities in the United States spent $83.7 billion for research and development. Sixty-four percent of applied biomedical research funding comes from within the industry itself, and 22 percent comes from the federal government, most often funded by grants from the NIH.

The diversity numbers are dismal at the top leadership level of these huge players in American health care. Ninety-two percent of 182 biotech and pharma companies are led by men. With the retirement of Kenneth Frazier, former CEO of Merck, there are no Black CEOs of a major pharmaceutical company. Universities are faring better, with more minorities and women in the top leadership roles, but those numbers are still disproportional to their membership in our society. White Americans represent 57.8 percent of the population. Hispanic and Latino Americans make up 18.7 percent of the population, and African Americans make up 12.1 percent. This country is 51 percent female. We can't afford to ignore this imbalance in representation in the institutions that wield so much power. Leaders of pharmaceutical companies and universities decide where money is allocated and what research is needed. That requires real diversity in organizations, especially at the top, to combat racial and cultural bias.

The financial power of the pharma-academic complex is an invasive element in American health care. Its positive power enables the growth of life-saving research, but it is shaded by the negativity of the bias in many of its branches.

CHAPTER 16

Payment Systems
as an Invasive
Health-Care Influence

HEALTH-CARE PAYMENT SYSTEMS MATTER. They contribute to health-care inequity, dividing our country into the haves and the have-nots. If you have money and great insurance, you can receive personalized health care focused on preventing and diagnosing diseases before they become untreatable. If you have less money and less-great insurance, you are less likely to get preventative care and more likely to receive delayed diagnosis and treatment. The people who are most subject to bias in this country are the most likely to have inadequate insurance, so their insurance payment systems wield immense power over who gets equitable health care in America.

Our country spends a huge amount of money on health care: four trillion dollars annually, 17.7 percent of GDP, the highest among developed countries. Ironically, our health outcomes fall far short of our spending. Our mature death rate and disease burden (the impact of a health problem as measured by financial cost, mortality, morbidity, or other indicators) is higher than in comparable countries. We rank last in health-care access and quality, indicating higher rates of amenable mortality than peer countries. Amenable mortality measures the rates of death considered preventable by timely and effective care. Clearly, throwing money at health care does not create better health-care outcomes.

What about the cost of health care for individuals and families? Annual family premiums for employer-sponsored health insurance topped $22,000 in 2021. On average, employees contributed $5,969 toward the cost of family coverage, with employers paying the rest. Ninety-two percent of covered workers had deductibles, and individuals on an average paid $1,669 a year out of pocket. Remember, these are averages. Many people pay even higher amounts. These numbers do not include the costs to 11.4 million enrolled in the state marketplaces and HealthCare.gov, or those getting Medicare or Medicaid. Additionally, twenty-eight million Americans do not have any health insurance at all.

Close to 30 percent of insured adults have postponed or canceled their medical care because they couldn't afford it, and 66.5 percent of bankruptcies were caused by high medical bills combined with the loss of work income due to illness. Savings and retirement accounts are rapidly depleted by thousands of dollars of treatment costs for a catastrophic or chronic disease. For those living paycheck to paycheck, medical costs can be even more devastating—homelessness, hunger, and loss of hope.

How Patients Perceive Payment Systems

Numerous studies report that the majority of Americans believe they are paying too much for their health care relative to its quality. They blame pharmaceutical companies, insurance companies, and hospitals, but it's hard to vent their anger and frustration on those faceless institutions. Instead, health-care providers often take the heat of patients' financial frustration. The angry patient brings their financial complaints to an office visit, though the provider has virtually no say in pricing decisions.

You can hear patient frustration in comments in our Pulse Survey:

> If I do not follow a doctor's treatment instructions, the reason most often is because I cannot afford to.

> Some of their treatment instructions require more money than I'm willing to spend.

> Meds too costly despite insurance.

> I have trouble losing weight, and I can't always afford recommendations that aren't covered by insurance.

One of our respondents was particularly upset:

> I could tell several stories, going back decades, about medical professionals who determined the care they would give me based on how much money they could make. If they could not make money, they either refused to provide care or provided only limited care. My experience has been that income—more than "race" or gender—determines care. A wealthy, African American woman is guaranteed to get better care than a poor, White male. If the book you are writing focuses on "race" and gender rather than income, then your book will not provide accurate information, nor will it address the main problems with health care: it costs too damn much, and most health-care *professionals* are in it for the money. Wealthy people—"race" and gender notwithstanding—get better health care than poor people.

I agree that individuals living in poverty get worse care than rich people, and the research backs us up. But I do not believe that doctors prescribe a treatment based on how much they expect to get paid. Are there some bad eggs among us? Of course. But the vast majority of doctors prescribe the treatment that they believe will get their patient better quicker and with the fewest complications.

Kathy recently had an incident with a prescription. The specialist had taken her history and prescribed a medication that she knew had good results and would not cause problems. When Kathy went to fill the prescription, her pharmacist said that it would cost five hundred dollars for a month's supply and suggested that she contact the doctor about other options. Within a day, the physician assistant had another drug for her at the cost of fifteen dollars a month. "I think the specialist was trying to do the right thing but was clueless to the actual cost of the medication," Kathy said. "I was grateful for the intervention on the part of my pharmacist. It made me hyperaware, however, that I had the background and skills to advocate for myself. I worry about those people who do not."

Her story leads me to the other issue with payment systems: They are too complicated and difficult for most patients to understand. In fact, they are often too complicated and difficult for most doctors to understand. In Kathy's example, the doctor had no idea how much the drug would cost Kathy because insurances vary so much on how much they cover for what drugs. In fact, most patients and doctors do not know what their insurers will pay for medical procedures. This leads to patients' distrust of doctors, and medical practices spending huge amounts of time communicating with insurance companies and explaining costs to patients.

Medical Billing 101

Let me take you into the back office of my practice, so you understand how medical billing works. A medical practice is a small business. Like any small business, I have overhead expenses such as payroll, supplies, equipment, and rent. My revenue comes from fees for services I perform for my patients. But unlike most small businesses, my revenues for the same service vary widely from one payer to another. I have a negotiated rate from each insurer, and each insurer can have a different fee schedule for each of the hundreds of services I provide.

What patients don't understand is that while they pay a lot of money to their health insurance company, the health insurance companies don't pay doctors very much at all. A primary care doctor like myself may be paid one hundred dollars for a standard physical. I may see that patient in person only once a year for their annual physical, but I incur costs for them throughout the year, when they call our office for refills or to ask questions. Then there's the administrative cost for that patient's record keeping, billing, and collections. That one hundred dollars I get for that patient once a year is quickly eaten up by all these costs. I'm certainly not making a profit on this patient.

For the patient paying thousands of dollars a year for insurance, they feel they are not getting value. Then they have high deductibles and additional costs for services and prescriptions not covered by insurance. They are surprised and often angry when they get a bill or learn that a service they request is uncovered. I can't tell you the number of times I have heard, "I don't see why I have to pay for this. I have good insurance!" You can see that this system doesn't work, either as a business model for me financially or for customer satisfaction.

Patients also don't realize that the insurance company does not pay the provider the retail price. With their big-company bargaining power they have set a lower price that they are willing to pay, and the provider has no choice but to accept that partial payment. The insurance reimbursement rarely covers the provider's costs.

Medical billing is complicated for both the patient *and* the doctor. If you have ever been hospitalized, you know what I am talking about. You received multiple bills for multiple services from multiple providers. Many of those statements had very little detail or codes that made no sense. Most medical billing statements were designed for third-party payers like insurance companies. They were never designed for consumers. Few patients can figure out a medical bill. They don't know if the hospital stay was two thousand or two hundred dollars per day. And how much of the charges will be covered by insurance? Does any other industry keep the consumer so out of the loop about actual costs?

For health-care providers, it is equally confusing. Each insurance company pays a different amount for each service. One insurance company may pay one hundred dollars for a physical, while another may pay seventy-five dollars. We are reimbursed set amounts for services we need to provide, such as an EKG or urine tests. Each of these charges has a different billing code and a different reimbursement from the insurers, and these differ not just by insurer but also by different plans from the same insurer. At the time we are delivering the medical service, we don't know what that patient's insurance is going to pay or not cover. So when a patient asks us what the service will cost them, we just have to make our best guess.

Each medical establishment contracts with each insurance company for an agreed-upon fee schedule for each of that insurance company's plans. Each fee schedule is specific to that practice, that company, and that plan. It would make sense for practices to cooperate in their negotiations with insurance companies, but there are antitrust laws throughout the country that prevent doctors from sharing their fee schedules with other practices.

It's an unnecessarily complicated numbers game. We have to process all these different charges and negotiate payment day in and day out. Many providers have to hire additional help just to make sure that the insurance companies are paying us the agreed-upon amounts. We often need to hire billing and collection agencies, which charge us between 3 and 6 percent of what we collect.

This isn't a problem just for independent health-care providers like my practice. Large health-care systems have the same challenges with revenue cycle management (RCM). But their size gives them more revenues to help pay for their RCM and higher revenue overall to offset costs. The bigger systems have multiple revenue streams: employed physicians, laboratory tests, physical therapy, radiology, outpatient surgery, inpatient hospital admissions, and even facilities charges. We small practices have only insurance reimbursements as revenue.

Because of obsolete antitrust laws, independent practitioners like myself are viewed as competitors and prohibited from joining in collective bargaining with insurance companies. Large health-care systems are considered single entities, which means they can negotiate fees that are up to 300 percent higher than what independent practices get. With that obvious economy of scale, it's not surprising that independent physician practices are increasingly consolidating. They just cannot afford to stay in business alone.

Big Money, Big Players

The health-care industry is massive, with many different players. For this discussion, I will focus on those organizations that directly provide health-care services and insurers who serve as third-party payers, not on others such as pharmaceutical, biotech, and medical technology companies. They are all money-making organizations, no matter whether they operate as for-profit or nonprofit entities. In fact, the majority of large health-care providers and insurers are run as nonprofit entities, but "not-for-profit" can be a misleading term. The major difference between nonprofits and for-profits is that nonprofits do not distribute their profits to private individuals. They still can make lots of money and reward their executives handsomely. Like any business focused on profits and saving money, they also need to manage costs. Sometimes, that means denying tests, MRIs, and certain treatments, which often puts them directly in conflict with the needs of doctors and patients. But those big managed-care care systems hold the purse strings. They have the big-business political and regulatory clout to determine who gets what health care.

The landscape has radically changed for medicine in America. Small hospitals have joined massive health systems. Practices have been purchased by hospitals. Insurers and providers have consolidated into managed-care organizations. This upheaval has changed health-care delivery for both doctors and patients. According to the American Medical Association, less than half of the doctors in this country now work in private practice. In 1983 more than 75 percent of physicians owned their own practices. By 2018, that number had dropped to 47 percent. Patients now have fewer choices of places to seek care. They find themselves being processed by medical "factories" where the doctors are production workers and the patients are products of the assembly line.

This shift to big-box medical care has not resulted in better health care for patients. Numerous studies report worse patient experiences and no significant reductions in hospital readmission or mortality rates. Only 13 percent of doctors agree that hospital employment of physicians is likely to enhance quality of care and decrease costs. The American Medical Association, which had previously advocated for consolidation with the hope of increased efficiency and improved patient care, has now launched an initiative to support private practices.

While the bigger-is-better consolidation strategy is not new to American health care, three recent policy changes have increased its momentum: the Affordable Care Act, changes in Medicare reimbursements, and regulation requiring electronic health record systems (EHRs).

The goals of the 2010 Affordable Care Act were to make affordable health insurance available to more people, to expand the Medicaid program to cover more people living in poverty, and to support medical-care-delivery methods that would lower health-care costs. While ACA has several benefits—particularly for those who previously could not afford health-care coverage or had preexisting conditions that caused them to be denied medical insurance—it has also caused financial challenges. Insurance companies need money from everyone to subsidize the small portion of Americans who account for the majority of health spending. In 2019, 5 percent of the population was responsible for nearly half of all health spending with an average of $61,000 in health expenditures annually, and the top 1 percent spent more than $130,000 per year. The bottom 50 percent of the population accounted for only 3 percent of all health spending with an average of $374.

At the same time, the aging population has increased demands on Medicare's resources, resulting in cuts to Medicare reimbursement to private practices. Of course, these cuts are meant to extend the resources of the system that so many depend on, but Medicare believed—and still believes—that bigger is better. Big hospital systems have more resources to negotiate rates with Medicare. They also receive higher rates for drugs and services than private practices. Private practices suffer from being small.

While electronic record keeping has provided patients access to their records and increased efficiency in doctors' offices, it comes with a high price. Physicians spend about twenty hours a week entering data into electronic records and complying with other documentation regulations. This documentation work distracts from patient care, and the time is uncompensated and is becoming a major factor in the high incidence of physician burnout. The business burden of electronic documentation is one reason why doctors decide to give up their own practices to become employees of hospitals.

Let me be clear that I am a physician *and* an entrepreneur. I believe in private practice and autonomy for physicians and patients. What I do not believe, however, is that big is always better when it comes to health care. In fact, I would argue that the American bias in favor of "bigger is better" has made practicing medicine much less fulfilling for doctors, has not led to the anticipated efficiencies, and, most important, has not improved patient outcomes. I particularly like a quote from Devorah Goldman, a visiting fellow at the Ethics and Public Policy Center, "... the replacement of the small doctor's office with large-scale facilities hasn't made medicine cheaper or access to it easier. It threatens to remove a core advantage of the small, privately owned practice: the sense of personal, immediate responsibility between the physician and patient."

Implications for Patients

Not only are patients paying more for health care with higher premiums and deductibles, but they now have less time with health-care providers. The only way for private practices to stay afloat is to see more patients, which means less time for individual appointments. Physicians in large health-care systems have the same challenge since they need to meet the productivity requirements of their employers. The high-speed medical interaction favors younger, affluent, White patients with high medical literacy, fewer risk factors, fewer communication barriers, and instant access to medical information on the internet. But what about individuals with disabilities or seniors, who may have multiple health issues? What about people from other cultures, who may speak different languages and need more time? What about people with medical mistrust or hesitancy because of negative past experiences with race or gender bias? These are the people most at risk in a system where their time with the doctor is limited.

The time problem can be somewhat alleviated by delegation of tasks within the health-care team. The doctor can delegate some patient interactions to other professionals, such as physician assistants and nurse practitioners. These days, physicians do not often call patients with test results; they rely on their support teams to extend their reach. Let's face it—Dr. Marcus Welby and his house calls don't exist anymore. The team-delegation model does have the downside of fracturing the one-on-one physician-patient relationship, and we know the strength of that relationship is important to the health of the patient. That's particularly true for the baby boomer generation, who grew up with Marcus Welby, or at critical periods in life like having a baby, raising children, or coping with a disease.

The groups who face bias are the least likely to have the time or money for preventative care, which is critical in minimizing risk factors for major diseases. Our current system puts very limited resources into preventative measures. It is focused on the acute diseases of here and now, not whether a person may develop diabetes in ten years or even if a current diabetes patient will develop complications in five years. Some insurers have tried to address this issue by instituting quality incentive programs where they share savings with doctors if they are able to save the insurer money and reach certain quality goals. At the end of the year, whatever money is saved is shared with the doctor. This should be a win-win for everyone, but unfortunately it doesn't always work that way. One reason is that the patient is not part of the reward equation. They are not incentivized to work toward better health outcomes. Another reason is that people fall through the cracks. For example, if a person has a high A1C (a diabetes warning marker) but feels fine, they probably come don't come to see me. I get points from the insurer because the cost of the patient is low, so I am saving them money. But then I get dinged on the patient because I haven't met quality criteria, which is to help prevent them from getting diabetes. So there goes the shared savings, which would have been helpful to keep my practice thriving.

Preventative care can also be ignored when a health insurance plan is using a formula based solely on current costs. We found a diabetes program that worked really well for our patients, but some were denied coverage because the cost of their prescription medications was currently too low to justify the cost of the program. The insurer did not want to fund a program that would cost more than what they were currently spending on each patient. Even though the program would have helped prevent later complications from diabetes and potentially reduce patients' medication needs, the insurance company did not approve coverage for many qualified patients. The insurers did not want to invest in these patients now, even though long-term they would probably have to pay more for those patients as their disease got worse. By the way, we were dinged in the end of year shared-savings calculation because of these patients, whose diabetes numbers were not in control, because we missed the quality requirements.

Two Ideas to Improve Payment Systems

There are ways we can improve how we pay for health care and also reduce bias and the inequities of our current system. Remember that this is a complex problem, so all ideas have pros and cons. But I still believe that we need major changes if we are to succeed in our goals of removing bias from health care and providing people with health care that maintains their right to be treated with respect and dignity. First, we need to guide people to use the lowest-cost point of entry in the health-care system, which is primary doctors. Under earlier managed-care systems, the primary doctor was the referral point to specialists. Customer protest has persuaded many insurance companies to remove that rule. Now, if your knee hurts you can directly call an orthopedic surgeon, who is much more expensive than a primary care doctor. More education is needed about the proper use of the ER and urgent care so people understand what types of disorders are urgent or an emergency. Urgent care costs the health-care system twice as much as a primary visit. Going to a specialist costs five to eight times as much, and going to the emergency room, ten times as much. As a consumer, you probably aren't aware of the cost differences. But the overall cost of health care would be much less if you took your medical problem to a primary care doctor first, freeing up more resources in the health-care system for programs directed at those most in need.

The primary care doctor can also provide continuity and comprehensive care for the patient. A primary care doctor looks at the whole person. Maybe that painful knee is related to some other underlying condition. An orthopedic specialist would focus on just the knee, but a primary doctor looks at your total heath. Taking your whole self, not just your knee, to the primary care doctor not only makes economic sense; it makes good long-term health sense.

Unfortunately, we have a huge primary doctor shortage that will only become worse. The high cost of medical school pushes students toward higher-paying specialties. Many potential primary doctors cannot deal with the economic stress of opening a practice, along with the grueling workload. If we are going to enact the primary care strategy for the sake of patients and our society, we need to subsidize the training and residency of primary care candidates.

Second, we need to push for transparency in medical billing and insurance coverage. Some patients ask me to check every aspect of their health at every visit. They want tests and blood work that are not medically necessary. When I let them know that their insurance company will not cover it, they say never mind. They know they are paying a fixed amount every month for their insurance, so they want to get the most out of it. That's just natural, but they don't know what their insurance will really cover. People don't know what they are looking at in their insurance policies and medical bills. They don't know how to read a bill, with its array of diagnosis codes and medical terms. They are shocked by surprise billing. Hospitals and doctors are often blamed for this, but often that bill is a surprise because the patient does not know what the insurance company covers. Sometimes, large health-care systems will give an estimate of what a procedure will cost and authorize that. If the final cost comes in higher, the health system explains, "That was just an estimate. As we discussed, you are responsible for the rest of the bill." Many people don't have the ability to pay those out-of-pocket costs, even when negotiated into monthly payments. We have effectively expected patients to be able to write a blank check for their health care. Whatever costs insurance doesn't cover become the patient's responsibility, often without warning of what the price will be. We call this surprise billing. This is a problem with insurance coverage transparency and should not be blamed on the doctor or health system. In another type of surprise billing, hospitals and health systems charge "out of network" fees after services have been rendered, which are often not covered by insurance. Patients who receive these bills are often shocked and unprepared, especially since most patients already pay a fortune for health insurance.

These payment system issues have wreaked havoc on our health-care system, causing frustration and burnout among physicians and financial stress to the patients. Patient care has suffered. The current health-care-payment system is like an invasive plant, crowding out our goals of good patient care and physician effectiveness from the troubled garden that is our current health-care system.

PART 4

A Prescription to Fix Health Care

I'm no longer accepting the things I cannot change... I'm changing the things I cannot accept.

—ANGELA DAVIS

CHAPTER 17

What We Must Do Now

WE ALL KNOW THE EXPRESSION "It takes a village to raise a child." It will take our whole village to bring equity to our health-care system: Health-care providers and their teams, patients, medical schools, policy makers, insurers, researchers, and government agencies. Each stakeholder in the health-care system can take practical steps to reduce the effects of bias. These are all doable. The solutions are within our reach.

What Can Health-Care Providers Do?

If you are a health-care provider feeling burnout as most of us are, you have probably found yourself sliding into quick but biased decision-making just to get the job done. First, take care of yourself. Don't become a casualty of the pandemic, along with the many of us who have left health care. Take a break to remember why you're here. It's all about the patients, in all their complexity, diversity, and individual differences. They're what makes our lives difficult, but also makes our work worthwhile. We need to treat them and ourselves as individuals. I have recommended ten things health providers and systems can do now:

1. **Diversity, equity, and inclusion training.** Every health-care system should use a standardized tool to assess health-care workers' attitudes about diverse populations. Since most bias is unconscious, formal assessment can help us see where there are issues and deficits. After bias is identified (and it almost always is), we must provide diversity, equity, and inclusion training before we send our workers out to care for a diverse patient population. It takes a humble and understanding spirit to treat our most vulnerable patients, and humility can be learned.

2. **Communication skill building for the health-care team.** Compassion, empathy, and humility training help build trust. We need to:

   • Make eye contact. Turn away from the computer and look at your patients. Consider using medical scribes for clinical documentation so providers can focus more on making a human connection with the patient.

   • Show respect by addressing patients by Mr./Mrs./Ms. plus their last name, unless they instruct you otherwise. A well-intentioned provider will often call a patient by their first name, but most African American patients prefer being addressed more formally. Ask the patient how they would like to be addressed and note that in their file.

   • Use touch according to the patient's preference. We will sometimes place a hand on the patient's shoulder or upper arm to communicate sincerity, but make sure your patient is comfortable with that sort of physical contact outside of the hands-on physical exam.

   • Ask the patient about their concerns. "Is there anything that you'd like to talk about today?"

   • Find out if there are social issues in your patient's life. "Do you have enough food to eat in your household?" or

"Do you worry about eviction?" Be prepared with information on available community resources.

- Always make sure to ask, "Do you have any questions today?"

3. **Survey, survey, survey.** Much like customer satisfaction surveys in business, patient surveys help health systems know how patients feel about their care and identify opportunities for better engagement and growth. Patient satisfaction surveys should follow every visit and be analyzed with reference to patient outcomes. Poor outcomes are often tied to patient dissatisfaction, because dissatisfied patients disengage from the health-care process. We should also ask how we can make the individual patient experience better. Use techniques suitable for your patients' communication needs. Some patients may not have a home computer or internet and may require a phone call or in-person survey. Some may require translation.

4. **Post community resource phone numbers in exam and waiting rooms.** These help patients know that you care about their well-being.

- Domestic/Intimate Partner Violence hotlines.
- Behavioral and mental-health referral sources for counseling services.
- Social service agencies (WIC program, food stamps, etc.).
- Community food banks.
- Suicide hotline phone numbers.
- Transportation resources.
- Information about HIV/AIDS resources and anonymous STD testing.

5. **Public service announcements.** Publish or broadcast public service announcements (posters, emails, videos, etc.) that show your practice as patient-centric and genuinely

concerned with the individual. If you use model patient photos, they should represent the population you serve.

6. **Effective use of support staff.** The shortage of physicians and their time constraints leaves patients feeling short-changed in follow-up care, but our support staff can fill in these gaps. Use community health workers, nurses, medical assistants, midwives, or doulas to make follow-up appointments, and make check-in calls to patients after their visits to see how they are doing and to remind them of upcoming appointments. Let your patients know that they may hear from all members of their care team, and that you are indeed one team.

7. **Reward providers and staff who perform well on patient satisfaction.** Beyond rewards for academic or financial performance, incentivize team members who perform well on patient satisfaction surveys. Let them know that patients' feelings count.

8. **Use anecdotal stories to motivate patients.** Many vulnerable individuals respond better to human stories or spiritual and natural examples than to medical statistics. For example, you might share a story about a patient you lost to a stroke because they did not take their blood pressure medicine. This personal approach may work better than informing that patient of their statistical risk of stroke. Make sure to tell the story with empathy: "I don't want that to happen to you, so please try to take your medication consistently."

9. **Incentivize patients to improve their health.** Incentivize patients with perks like gift cards for flu shot participation. (Be careful not to violate Stark laws.) For years I have offered a free lunch to anyone who believes they contracted the flu from the flu shot. I share with my patients that no one has ever had to take me up on that lunch offer, and that gives them comfort in accepting the flu shot. Or you could have

a staff silly-costume day where the entire team dresses up if they do not reach a certain patient compliance goal.

10. **Create a patient advisory council that reflects the community.** Ask a group of key patients to represent their peers in advising your team on how you could better serve them.

What Can Patients Do?

1. **Get the COVID vaccine and booster.** This is your best protection against getting seriously ill or dying. My practice has a great COVID vaccination adoption rate, consistently more than twenty points above the national average. As of December 2021, over 17 percent of U.S. adults remained unvaccinated, causing over 690,000 preventable COVID-19 hospitalizations. So far, the cost of care for preventable illness in unvaccinated patients is over $13 billion dollars. Vaccines should be mandated, perhaps through insurance coverage: Insurers could give no choice but to get vaccinated or lose coverage. Vaccine mandates could also be enforced through the workplace or as a requirement to enter public places.

2. **Seek your care from primary care and/or urgent care.** When a patient's first stop for non-emergent medical care is at the emergency room, the cost of care skyrockets. Avoid the ER unless it truly is an emergency. Taking your UTI to the ER can cost ten times the cost of treating it in a primary care or urgent care setting. Of course, this means that patients should have a primary care physician on record. Many do not.

3. **Understand that your doctor is just one member of your health-care team.** Get comfortable seeing PAs, NPs, or RNs for routine issues. Understand that there is a shortage of doctors, especially in primary care, and other care team

members are qualified to work with you. This may mean speaking with a nurse or medical assistant about test results or accepting that you may not be able to speak directly with your doctor without an appointment.

4. **Be gracious to your health-care workers.** Please be kind to your health-care providers, especially now, as we have all been traumatized by the demands of the COVID-19 pandemic. Know that we are overworked, understaffed, and doing the best we can to be gracious to you. You can do the same for us.

What Can Medical Schools Do?

1. **Share stories on the human condition.** Much of medical training is about science, but these days you also hear of courses like Columbia's in narrative medicine: "... an interdisciplinary field that brings powerful narrative skills of radical listening and creativity from the humanities and the arts to address the needs of all who seek and deliver health care. It enables patients and caregivers to voice their experience, to be heard, to be recognized, and to be valued, improving the delivery of health care. This evolving transdisciplinary field of enquiry addresses issues of structural inequality and social justice in health care."

Sounds right up our alley, right? Voices of patients and caregivers addressing structural inequality and social justice in health care? That's what we're talking about.

2. **Teach cultural humility as part of diversity, equity, and inclusion training.** Further, teach sensitivity to non-ethnic issues such as age, disability status, and weight.

3. **Require rotations in underserved areas.** They need doctors, and medical students need to be exposed to the kinds of patients they will need to serve.
4. **Admit more qualified Black and Brown students.** As well as those from disadvantaged backgrounds and rural areas.
5. **Make all medical students feel included in the medical community.** Build your medical school into an inclusive community. Offer more individually tailored personal and academic support to ensure successful completion of the curriculum. Acknowledge their diversity as a strength.

What Can Policy Makers Do?

1. **Push legislation for more federally supported medical schools and residency training.** This is urgent. We have a deficit of physicians in the United States already, and more than two in five working physicians will reach retirement age in the next decade. In addition, we expect the patient population to grow by another 10 percent, with a 42 percent increase in those over sixty-five. We need more doctors now, but we will desperately need more doctors in the future. The cost of medical school is beyond the financial reach of many qualified students. Medical education needs federal support.
2. **Hold insurance companies accountable.** Insurance companies should invest more into primary care infrastructure. They should be more transparent in their billing processes for both patients and doctors. We need legislation to prevent "surprise" medical bills and to prevent illegitimate denials of medical services by insurers. Opaque insurance reimbursement processes cause the average medical practice to spend up to 10 percent of its revenue on billing and collection, which is much more than in other industries.

3. **Encourage use of patient-centered medical home (PCMH) models.** Policy should require insurance companies to operate more transparently in their reimbursement of PCMH practices. Many current quality-metric reward schemes are overly complicated, making it difficult for practices to implement the PCMH.

4. **Make health insurance companies nonprofit.** Many insurance companies are for-profit, which means that their primary stakeholders are their stockholders, not the medical system or its patients. The health insurance industry pays its CEOs seven- or eight-figure salaries, while primary care practices struggle just to keep their doors open, and doctors' salaries have remained stagnant for decades.

5. **Reduce the allowed percentage of claims denied by insurance companies.** One in five insurance claims is denied, with a wide variation in denial rates among the insurers. Some insurers deny very few claims, while others deny payment for as much as 45 percent of claims. Medical facilities can appeal those denials, but smaller medical facilities often do not have the means to pursue payment. Often healthcare systems cannot not afford to appeal, so unpaid claims add to the insurers' bottom line and to the medical system's losses. These claim denials do not usually get passed on as the patients' payment responsibility, but I am sure that most patients do not realize that their doctor is taking a loss on their treatment. Policy changes should regulate the percentage of claims that an insurance company can deny.

What Can Insurers Do?

In the United States, insurers hold the purse strings for the entire health-care system. How insurance companies are managed effects the care delivery system all the way down the line. Insurers need to optimize their efficiency of operations and efficacy of service delivery.

1. **Pay providers and hospitals on time.**
2. **Remove barriers to payments.** Reduce denial rates and equalize those rates across payers. Some denials are legitimate, as when the patient's identity cannot be verified due to registration errors or policy name variations. But some insurers encourage denials purely to up their bottom line. These are unjustified.
3. **Incentivize providers for good care and good outcomes.** Not just for saving costs. Our practice participates in incentive programs that offer us additional payments for saving money for the health insurance company and meeting quality goals. These models should decouple rewards for saving money from those that reward for achieving quality metrics.

What Can Researchers Do?

Medical research is essential to promote quality improvements and innovation in health care. Historically, there has been a lack of diversity (gender, racial/ethnic, and age) of subjects in clinical trials. Even when there is diverse representation, the results have not always been analyzed by race, ethnicity, or gender.

1. **Work harder to include more women and minorities in clinical research.** Prior to 1993, most researchers treated women essentially the same as men in clinical research. Thanks to the NIH Revitalization Act of 1993, which mandates inclusion of women and minorities in clinical research, we now have more representation, but we need

more medical research studies exclusively on women and minority populations.

2. **We need more education and outreach to historically excluded and misused populations.** We have a long way to go to build trust in minority populations who have a history of maltreatment by medical research. Researchers need to be transparent about their medical research methods and goals, target their communications to specific populations, and build in incentives for minorities' participation. Researchers should work to better understand research hesitation in certain populations so that we can better target their concerns and create a more inclusive clinical research community.

3. **Do more research into the patient experience and its relationship with medical mistrust.** Medical providers are mystified by the level of mistrust they face in their patients. We need to understand where that mistrust is rooted in the patients' experience with the medical system. We need to study the patient-medical-system interaction itself. How do patients see us? In what ways has our communication broken down to the point of mistrust? How can we face our patients with better cultural sensitivity? These are essential questions for communication research.

What Can Advocacy Groups Do?

Patient advocacy groups fall into three categories: government, nonprofit, and for-profit. I will focus here on the government advocacy groups, including: the Centers for Disease Control, U.S. Department of Health and Human Services, the National Institutes of Health, the Food and Drug Administration, and the Agency for Healthcare Quality Research.

1. **Maintain a non-political position.** Watching the process of passing of the Affordable Care Act was my first experience of polarizing and politicized medical legislation. "Obamacare" marked the beginning of a political conversation about who should pay for health care, raising some essential questions: Is health care a right or a privilege? Should insurance be mandated? But that conversation should not be polarized along political lines. These questions should address fundamental ethical and economic issues, not party affiliations.

2. **Agree on this issue: Health care is a right.** All individuals should be afforded basic human rights. The United Nations Universal Declaration of Human Rights Article 25 addresses health care: "Everyone has the right to a standard of living adequate for the health and well-being of himself and of his family, including food, clothing, housing and medical care and necessary social services, and the right to security in the event of unemployment, sickness, disability, widowhood, old age or other lack of livelihood in circumstances beyond his control." The United Nations has declared medical care to be a basic human right. No matter our political affiliation, can't we all work toward agreeing on just that?

3. **Advocate for a universal health-care system.** The U.S. remains the only developed country without universal health care. Approximately 8.6 percent of the population are without health insurance despite the efforts of the Affordable Care Act. We can restructure our health-care system to offer universal coverage for basic care without overburdening the economy. Those of us with insurance have our payments increased to subsidize the uninsured, so we end up paying for their more costly episodes of care. Government agencies need to join the fight for universal health care.

4. **Make health literacy information more available.** Government agencies should continue to promote health literacy. Patients need to be educated on their rights to fair treatment, confidentiality, and informed consent. Education materials should be tailored to their audiences, considering our population's diversity of language and culture, as well as their native-language literacy challenges. Patients need to be taught to be critical consumers of health information.

5. **Advocate for measures to ban misinformation.** Special interests are cranking out reams of medical misinformation, often under the protection of "freedom of speech." Patient advocacy organizations need to intervene against this dangerous flow of false health information. Some misinformation campaigns even have overseas sources, as with the Russian troll factories that spread COVID vaccine misinformation.

6. **Government agencies should not allow political pressure to shape their medical advice to the public.** When organizations like the CDC are influenced by political pressure, it erodes public trust and ultimately harms our health. Recent U.S. history shows examples of political interference from both sides of the aisle: According to a House panel on the coronavirus response, there was evidence that the Trump administration carried out a pressure campaign to force changes to government scientific publications for political purposes. Under the Biden administration as well, the CDC was evidently pressured to reduce required quarantine from ten to five days, in spite of the lack of supporting evidence or vetting of the new policy by other government agencies.

7. **Advocate for health equity.** Patient advocacy agencies should work toward reducing health disparities by advocating for and educating our most vulnerable patients. We need evidence-based health education with emphasis on

preventative care beginning in elementary schools. Health education needs to address bias, inclusion, and health equity issues.

8. **Mandate a basic level of science education on scientific facts, methods, and principles.** Science education needs to be relevant and engaging, encouraging more children to consider careers in medicine and health careers.

9. **Root out anti-science bias.** Anti-science sentiment is now so strong as to threaten the health of our nation, persuading people to ignore or distrust the life-saving advances that science has made over the past century. This links back to our earlier calls to depoliticize health information and improve science education.

CHAPTER 18

Changing the Future of Health Care in America

OVER THE PAST TWO CENTURIES, we have come a long way in medical innovation, advancements, and extending life expectancy. Progress had been steady until the global COVID pandemic, which has eliminated some public health gains. The pandemic has erased 28 million potential human life–years around the globe. The year 2020 marked a huge step backward for health care.

How did the pandemic manage to push us backward? We will be asking that question for years to come. We will blame hospitals. We will blame health organizations. We will blame countries. We will blame the media. We will blame politics. We will blame science. We will blame ignorance. We will blame the supply chain. The list goes on. There may be some truth in each of them.

But I would like to suggest another reason: Dismissal. Just as we dismiss people because of their skin color, gender, age, weight, or disability, Americans have dismissed a health-care model that could improve life for many and protect us from inevitable future pandemics and global catastrophes. All the signs and experts' predictions point to a future where global warming will wreak havoc on our planet, endangering our food and water supplies and even the foundations of civilization. The environment will pay us back for our mistreatment, creating threats to human health. Our health-care system needs a structure and focus that will respect and protect the vulnerable before global chaos leaves the world only to the powerful. We need a health-care system that values and protects us all.

Here are seven conditions necessary for the strong, resilient health-care system we need for the future. Everyone would have basic health needs covered, we would rebuild the public's trust in health care, and we would close health disparity gaps to provide a long, healthy, balanced life for everyone.

I dream of a health-care system where:

- Everyone in America has health-care coverage and health-care access. These are basic human rights.
- Every patient feels validated and cared for regardless of race, ethnicity, disability, gender, age, or health history.
- The health-care team works together with the individual patient's welfare foremost, providing continuity of care, with communication among primary care providers, specialties, clinics, community, and home care providers, across the life span of every patient.
- The entire health-care system is free of the influences of politics and religion.
- We use smart technology to better plan and coordinate care and to strengthen the human connections in care delivery.
- Primary care can be specialized for historically vulnerable groups: women, minorities, individuals who identify as LGBTQIA, people with disabilities, seniors, immigrants, or the chronically ill.
- Doctors from diverse and historically vulnerable backgrounds will be recruited and supported in medical training and throughout their careers.

1: Embrace Health Care for All

Access to basic health-care coverage is a human right. There should be universal basic health-care coverage for all, regardless of a person's ability to pay. Basic coverage includes basic life-saving measures and chronic-disease management. We can fund it by redirecting money from current insurance premiums into a public health insurance pool. Universal coverage would still allow private insurance options for those who wish to purchase additional coverage for therapies not covered by a basic model.

Universal health care would require a consistent fee-for-service schedule, which could be adjusted for cost by locality, as with the current Medicare fee schedule. Within the same region, no two doctors should be paid differently for the same work. Currently, many states prohibit doctors from even sharing their fee schedules. Fair reimbursement rate and fee schedules require transparency, so all doctors at the same level can expect the same fees for each unit of the same service. This would also reduce the complexities now involved in billing and collections. It would eliminate the need for the adjustment process, which currently makes health care one of the most complex industries for revenue cycle management. Universal care, with its fair fee schedule, would also reduce the burgeoning administrative costs in health care.

To achieve universal health care, we must invest more in prevention and the "first line of defense" function of primary care. We need more primary care providers and more investment in their practices. Given the shortage of primary care doctors now and the huge gap anticipated in the future, we need to invest in federal, state, and local programs to subsidize medical school for those specializing in primary medicine. We should provide incentives to set up primary care practices in underserved urban and rural areas, providing access for many patients now without primary care and diverting them from the use of hospital ERs for primary care needs. Many programs in the United States encourage businesses and economic development in underserved areas, and those models can also be applied to health care.

By centralizing care in a "Patient Care Home" model, patients would become more accepting of their health-care providers as a team. The team works together to provide efficient continuity of care. The physician leads the patient's care team, with nurse practitioners, physician assistants, registered nurses, licensed practical nurses, and medical assistants to help with communication, care management, care coordination, and care delivery. The team model allows for more time with each patient according to need and allows the system to focus more on the patient and less on the business transaction. Finally, we need to include mental health in universal health coverage. Mental health providers should join primary practice teams, affirming the need for integrated mental and physical health services.

#2: Reduce Medical Bias and Health Inequity

Doctors from diverse and vulnerable backgrounds need to be recruited and supported. As a practicing physician who grew up Black and living in poverty, I have to say that my personal suffering has affected my work as a doctor more than my choice of medical school. Being a social outcast and victim of vitriolic bias made me humbler. Growing up in poverty made me more vulnerable and compassionate. Losing my infant son because of being dismissed by an arrogant doctor made me determined to make a difference.

We need more providers with diverse life experiences, those who can relate to our most vulnerable patients. I have personally attempted to make inroads there by forming a nonprofit, Premedical Explorers. After Dr. Susan Moore's death, some of my high school friends convened to discuss how we might pay homage to her life and legacy. We created a mentoring program for minority high school students to help prepare them for medical training, with the long-term goal of increasing the number of Black doctors. We started in our high school alma mater, with the plan to spread the program across the country over the next several years.

We need diverse medical school student bodies, residency programs, and health-care system leadership teams to ensure that diverse students are given a fair chance at admission. We need that diversity across the board, in every health-care unit in America, including hospitals, clinics, outpatient centers, private offices, home care teams, and beyond. Special effort is needed to bring diverse people into leadership positions where they would participate in decisions on policy, research, and medical innovation.

Bias will always exist, but antibias and cultural humility training will direct health-care providers toward bias-free diagnostic and treatment decisions. This training should begin in medical school and carry through residency and beyond, as a part of the regular continuing medical education (CME) required for all doctors and licensed health-care workers. Antibias training should be included right along with the requirements for clinical medical education. Medical board exams should cover this essential skill. The same model of education should be required for all members of the health-care team, including allied health professions. Further, we should create a new medical specialty aimed at diversity, equity, and inclusion, which would identify strategies to counteract the effects of disenfranchisement and bias.

Racism in health care is rooted in the structural racism of America. We cannot expect a reduction in medical racism while racism still runs rampant in our society. We must continue our social justice efforts with a goal of achieving equality and justice for all. We have to understand that the social determinants of health are more than just a statistical study, but can provide a framework for action on a societal level.

We should monitor for health outcome disparities, not just among racial groups but also among patients with disabilities, patients who are obese, our seniors, and individuals who identify as LGBTQIA. That's not hard to do: Modern data aggregation and analysis tools can analyze data by any variable or parameter we choose. Gaps in care should be tied to quality measures that are tied to reimbursement. Reimbursement and quality incentives should be tied to patients' reported experiences, reduction of health disparity gaps, and positive patient outcomes. The goal is to erase all health disparities for those vulnerable groups.

Disenfranchised patients will be able to trust the medical profession again when they feel accepted, validated, and cared for as individuals. We can form specialized primary care offices caring for focused patient groups, such as women, individuals who identity as LGBTQIA, individuals with disabilities, or those from non-mainstream cultures. I have seen this sort of segmentation among mental health therapists, who often list their areas of interest or specialization. Knowing our specialties, patients could choose the right providers for their needs.

#3 Remove Politics and Religion from Health Care

Vaccination and reproductive rights: two health-care issues that have fallen victim to the influence of politics and religion. America's political divide over vaccinations has harmed the nation's health. Prior to the pandemic, the anti-vax movement was based on perceived medical issues like rising rates of autism. Opinions on that issue are now tied to politics. Some people believe that vaccine mandates for COVID and other diseases take away their personal freedom. Medical experts fear that the growing number of political anti-vaxxers will lead to a surge in diseases like mumps, whooping cough, and smallpox, as well as COVID.

I have the same concern, while still trying to honor my patients' individual choices, but I believe we need to educate those choices with science-based educational programs starting in elementary school and extending into adulthood. We need communication training for primary doctors and pediatricians on how to talk with patients who are wary of vaccination. We can accept their right to think differently while still educating them with the facts.

The public needs to be educated on the importance of vaccinations to our society's health. We have had some success with prior public information campaigns, such as in the danger of drunk driving. Following a 1982 public information campaign that showed that drunk driving was a societal issue, drunk driving fatalities decreased 52 percent. Among persons under twenty-one, drunk driving fatalities have decreased 83 percent. While this has come about partially from increased legal penalties, public education has also helped reduce those numbers.

President Obama once said, "Nobody's pro abortion." I agree with him wholeheartedly. However, if a woman believes that abortion is the best option for her and her family, she has the right to control her own body, and abortion should be a legal choice. That individual decision should be free of influence from religious groups and government. We individuals should respect each other's opinions, allowing different people to make different choices. Women should have the freedom to act on their own beliefs about their own reproduction, without interfering with others' choices.

Politics and religion have found their way into publicly available information, making it hard for the average person to verify the source and validity of what they hear and read. We need to know where to find accurate health information free of political influence. We need a way of identifying and removing misinformation, perhaps a Snopes-like fact-checker for medical information.

Finally, we need to prevent lobbying and political contributions from influencing health-care policy. Pharmaceutical companies, insurers, health-care systems, and other players in the system spend hundreds of millions of dollars on lobbying and political financial influence. In fact, pharmaceutical and health-products companies and insurers are the top spenders on political influence for both Democrats and Republicans. Lawmakers cannot help but be swayed by those contributions, endangering the passage of fair health-care legislation.

#4: Improve Access to Smart Technology

Technology does great things for both patients and health-care providers. It helps us better coordinate care, improve patient engagement through digital communication and information sharing, and provides central access to medical records. Patients can now access their own records through patient portals. Telemedicine makes it possible for them to see a health-care provider without coming to the office.

The problem is that these benefits of technology currently reach only part of the American population. One in four households does not have access to home internet because of either location or cost. As we become more dependent on the internet for delivery of health-care services and information, we need to provide universal internet access. We need to provide tech training for our older population, who could most benefit from home access to health care. We need to ensure that our systems are user-friendly for individuals with disabilities.

Some digital technologies have inherited our human bias. I would like to use machine learning (AI) for prognostication and to enhance the patient experience, but some AI-driven software programs have been found to have bias, even some AI-driven bias detection programs. We must make sure that technology does not perpetuate the same bias as humans.

Finally, we need to lower the cost of diagnostic technology. Hospitals and imaging clinics charge between one and two thousand dollars for a single MRI scan. The cost of the equipment itself can run over a million dollars. Doctors fight insurers to pay for scans for their patients, or patients are asked to pay out of pocket, affordable only for the very rich. Technology needs to reduce, not increase, health-care inequity.

#5 Support Paid and Unpaid Caregivers

Our current health-care system has failed to consider caregivers—both unpaid and paid—as an essential part of the health-care system. Our population is aging, and the need for caregivers is growing. We can support unpaid caregivers with financial assistance, respite care, and teaching of self-care techniques. Paid caregivers need large pay increases. Many make less than minimum wage. Many are hired through private home-care agencies, so we need to look at the reimbursement model to make sure both employees and agency owners are being compensated fairly. We need to recognize all caregivers as vital contributors to maintaining the health of so many.

#6: Patients Must Acknowledge Their Responsibility

I encourage patients to treat their health-care teams with respect and appreciation. Patients need to recognize their own responsibilities in their health care and in their interactions with the health-care team. Yes, doctors do get weary and may not always have their patient interaction skills working as well as they should, but patients need to acknowledge that doctors and their teams are human, like them. We doctors are trying daily to remember the same of our patients.

COVID and its associated antiscience movement have had a demoralizing effect on our doctors and nurses. The life-and-death pressures of the pandemic have stretched us to our limit. The last straw for us, though, was seeing patients forming opinions about vaccination or medical treatment based on information from friends, family, and unvalidated internet sources, so devaluing our medical expertise and even science itself. Doctors do like to share decision-making with knowledgeable patients, but when patients dictate their own care based on "alternative facts," we doctors begin to wonder why we're here.

We give advice and treatment to heal you, but you can't heal unless you do the work to apply that advice and accept that treatment. Patient responsibility requires compliance with doctor recommendations. According to the National Institutes of Health, 75 percent of Americans have trouble taking their medicine as directed. Medical nonadherence costs the medical system millions of dollars and, more important, costs people their health. They have no problem turning their legal matters over to lawyers, taking an accountant's advice about taxes, or relying on a mechanic to fix their cars. With doctors, though, they often ignore our advice and don't follow through with prescribed treatment. The doctor-patient partnership is a 50–50 deal. Just imagine the frustration for health-care providers, whose only goal is to get people well, when patients won't take their half of the responsibility.

7: Practice Comprehensive Self-Care

One thing we have learned from research like the Blue Zone is that comprehensive self-care that includes actions to enhance physical, mental, emotional, and spiritual health can lead to a longer and healthier life. We can acknowledge that there are many things that are beyond our control, and we do not need to live in a place of blame bias. We can put faith in new technologies that enhance treatment and diagnosis and enable health care to be delivered more efficient and accessible ways. We can support the development of new vaccines, medications, and medical devices to handle terrible diseases. We can train health-care teams to operate with less bias and create policies that support our most vulnerable populations.

Yet, at the end of the day, we—both patients AND health-care providers—need to take personal responsibility to practice comprehensive self-care. We know the connection of anxiety, stress, and depression to physical ailments. We understand a life filled with exercise and a healthy diet can reduce heart disease, obesity, and cancer. We know that intellectual stimulation and connection to others keep our minds more vibrant. There are self-care strategies that most of us can put in place no matter what our economic situation, race, gender, sexual orientation, or age.

As Hippocrates, who is considered the father of medicine, said: "Healing is a matter of time, but it is sometimes also a matter of opportunity." Let's go seize the opportunity for self-care.

CHAPTER 19

Inclusion Leads to Life

I AM SITTING IN THE audience watching my daughter in her high school musical. She is the lead, and her voice and stage presence keep the audience mesmerized. Her poise and confidence shine through like a bright star. My daughter has been performing for ten years and never lets anything stop her from doing what she loves and doing it well. She never lets anyone dismiss her. My son also thrives. He recently pivoted his course of study in college, and I am so impressed by his resilience and perseverance. I especially applaud his courageousness in advocating for himself and not letting anyone dismiss him.

I am so proud of both of them. I think of myself at their ages and how the weight of poverty, race, and gender tried so hard to keep me down. I was surrounded by overt bias and prejudice and the microaggressions that are part of a Black person's life, no matter what their age. Did it make me stronger? Yes. Could it have pulled me down? An even bigger yes.

I am glad these are different times for my daughter and son. This is a better world for them in some ways. But I still worry intensely about their futures. I worry that when my extremely intelligent and articulate son leaves his house, he will be in danger because he is a Black man. I worry that my talented daughter will have doors closed because she is a Black woman. I know too well the statistics that say that my kids may not be diagnosed or treated adequately for certain diseases because of their skin color and gender. These fears are why I fight against prejudice and bias. I will not let the world dismiss my children.

Dismissal leads to death. I don't just mean literal loss of life, but also the death of the spirit, the death of dreams, the death of potential. Dismissal damages so many lives: a child with disabilities bullied at school, a worker excluded from a job because of race or gender, a beautiful body hidden in shame after disrespect in social media, a senior whose brilliant ideas are ignored because their hair is white. Each of these dismissals damages a human life. Sometimes that human manages to weld that damage into strength, but at other times we witness the destruction of a person and their potential.

Each of us is individually responsible for acting on behalf of all of us. In the words of Martin Niemöller, a German Lutheran pastor, writing in 1946:

> First they came for the socialists, and I did not speak out—because I was not a socialist.
> Then they came for the trade unionists, and I did not speak out—because I was not a trade unionist.
> Then they came for the Jews, and I did not speak out—because I was not a Jew.
> Then they came for me—and there was no one left to speak for me.

I was struck by two things in these poignant words. First, we must each take personal responsibility. Each of us is responsible for becoming an agent of change. Each of us needs to speak out. Each of us is responsible to become "woke." Second, universal inclusion means speaking out not only for your group, but for all groups. It means taking action to show that there are no "others"; there is only "we." Because if WE do not speak out, sooner or later THEY will come for us.

But let me take a deep breath, because at heart I am an optimist. Let me take a breath of hope. COVID raised our social consciousness of the wrongness of what we used to call "normal." We can't go back there. During our isolation, we learned what it feels like to be excluded, how lonely it is when we are not allowed to be part of a vibrant life. We are getting sick of the political divide in America and the vitriolic lies that clog our social media. We have woken up to the fact that millions are deprived of equitable health care. We have watched people die from ignorance and neglect. Health disparities are no longer just an academic and policy backroom discussion. We are more open to new ideas than before. Crisis is a powerful catalyst for change; now we must keep the momentum going.

Yes, I believe deeply that inclusion leads to life. I am a mother, wife, niece, cousin, and friend. I am a doctor who has taken an oath to heal to the best of my capabilities. I know one thing: Life is a blessing that we can never take for granted.

Request

If you would like to take action against the biases that undermine our health care, I urge you to donate to the Premedical Explorers Program, which provides Black youth with a premed learning program during the school year. Our goal is simple: 89,500 new Black doctors in ten years. Find us at https://premedexplorers.org/donate/.

Discussion Guide

1. Have you ever felt dismissed by a health-care professional? What was your reaction? After reading this book, do you think you would respond differently?
2. Did it surprise you to think of doctors as being vulnerable? If so, in what way would it change how you engage with your doctor and other health-care workers?
3. How have your experiences during the pandemic affected how your see the health-care system? What have been some of the positives and negatives?
4. We've talked about many different types of bias in this book. Explore the bias that has the most impact on your own life and how it has affected your physical and mental health.
5. What do you like about technology that is used in health care, such as computerized record-taking and portals? Have they enhanced your relationship with your doctor or taken away from the patient experience?
6. Do you believe that things like poverty and lack of food, education, transportation, and safe housing lead to different health outcomes for the haves and have-nots? If so, what issues would you want to see addressed to change the world?
7. Of the ideas posed to improve health care, what would you consider your top three immediate recommendations and your top three future recommendations?

8. If you could have a completely candid conversation with your doctor, what would you want to tell them about how you want to be treated?
9. If you could have a completely candid conversation with your patient, what would you want to tell them about how you want to be treated?
10. What surprised you the most in this book?
11. Did you find your opinion changed by any of the stories and information shared in this book? What and how?

Acknowledgments

Angela's Acknowledgments

I would like to thank and acknowledge my maternal grandmother, Mary Helen Cotton, a former nurse at a Michigan prison, who was affectionately called "Mother Love" by the inmates who adored her. She demonstrated my very first example of patient care that was unconditional and free from judgment. I am a better doctor because of her. I would also like to acknowledge Dr. Catherine Lucey, my first clinical preceptor, for graciously setting the bar for providing unbiased patient care with such love and compassion. Your shoes will never be filled, yet I hope you continue to share your gifts with more future doctors. I would also like to thank my loving husband for caring for and nurturing me, while I cared for and nurtured others. I am also so very grateful for my two beautiful children, who continue to make me happy and proud.

Kathy's Acknowledgments

I would like to thank my friends and family for their wisdom, skills, and support, particularly Jan Heyneman, Joe Edwardsen, Ben Edwardsen, Jordan Council, and Chris O'Brien. A special shout-out to my multigenerational household, who put up with a closed door and slightly grumpy wife, mother, and grandma during this all-encompassing project. Gratitude to my colleagues at goFirestarter, who picked up slack and constantly encouraged. Thanks to Leticia Gomez, literary agent extraordinaire, who believed that this book was as important as we did. Michaela Hamilton and her team from Kensington Publishing have offered amazing support and guidance. Most of all, I want to profoundly thank Dr. Angela Marshall, who is one of the most empathetic, listening, and respectful persons I have ever met.

Notes

1. How Dismissal Can Lead to Death

17   *A study published in the* New England Journal of Medicine: Elizabeth Nable, "Coronary Heart Disease in Women—An Ounce of Prevention," *New England Journal of Medicine* 343, no. 8 (August 2000): 572–74.

19   *Women in pain*: Laura Kiesel, "Women and Pain: Disparities in Experience and Treatment," *Harvard Health* (blog), Harvard Health Publishing, October 9, 2017, https://www.health.harvard.edu/blog/women-and-pain-disparities-in-experi ence-and-treatment-2017100912562.

20   *According to the* 2018 National Health: "2018 National Healthcare Quality and Disparities Report" (Rockville, MD: Agency for Healthcare Research and Qual- ity, 2019), https://www.ahrq.gov/sites/default/files/wysiwyg/research/findings/ nhqrdr/2018qdr-final-es.pdf.

20   *The Black infant mortality rate*: Danielle M. Ely and Anne K. Driscoll, "Infant Mortality in the United States, 2018: Data from the Period Linked Birth/Infant Death File," *National Vital Statistics Report* 69, no. 7 (July 16, 2020), Table 2, https://www.cdc.gov/nchs/data/nvsr/nvsr69/NVSR-69-7-508.pdf.

21–22   *As recently as 2016, in a study published*: Kelly M. Hoffman, Sophie Trawalter, Jordan R. Axt, and M. Norman Oliver, "Racial Bias in Pain Assessment and Treatment Recommendations, and False Beliefs About Biological Differences Between Blacks and Whites," *Proceedings of the National Academy of Sciences* 113, no. 16 (April 4, 2016): 4296–4301, https://doi.org/10.1073/pnas.1516047113.

22   *Additionally, a meta-analysis of twenty years of studies covering*: Salimah H. Meghani, Eeeseung Byun, and Rollin M. Gallagher, "Time to Take Stock: A Meta-Analysis and Systematic Review of Analgesic Treatment Disparities for Pain in the United States," *Pain Medicine* 13, no. 2 (February 2012): 150–74, https://doi.org/10.1111/j.1526-4637.2011.01310.x.

25   *I swear to fulfill*: "Medical Definition of Hippocratic Oath," medterms, Medicine Net, https://www.medicinenet.com/hippocratic_oath/definition.htm.

2. We're All Vulnerable

33   *In a January 2019 Pew Research Center survey*: Cary Funk, Meg Hefferon, Brian Kennedy, and Courtney Johnson, "Trust and Mistrust in Americans' Views of Scientific Experts," Pew Research Center, August 2, 2019, https://www.pew research.org/science/2019/08/02/trust-and-mistrust-in-americans-views-of -scientific-experts/.

34   *"Equity involves trying to understand"*: "Equity vs. Equality and Other Racial Justice Definitions," Annie E. Casey Foundation, April 14, 2021, https:// www.aecf.org/blog/racial-justice-definitions.

35   *The Centers for Disease Control and Prevention (CDC)*: "Health Disparities," Alzheimer's Disease and Healthy Aging, Division of Population Health, National Center for Chronic Disease Prevention and Health Promotion, Centers for Disease Control and Prevention, January 31, 2017, https://www.cdc.gov/ aging/disparities/index.htm#:~:text=Health%20disparities%20are%20pre ventable%20differences,other%20population%20groups%2C%20and%20co mmunities.

35   *The Office of Disease Prevention and Health Promotion (ODPHP) explains*: "Disparities," Office of Disease Prevention and Health Promotion, https://www. healthypeople.gov/2020/about/foundation-health-measures/Disparities.

39   *A recent study found that having an adequate*: "More Primary Care Physicians Could Mean Gains in Life Expectancy, Fewer Deaths," news release, EurekAlert!, American Association for the Advancement of Science, March 22, 2021, https://www.eurekalert.org/news-releases/488443.

39   *Dr. Sonali Mantoo, a critical care physician, explains*: Sonali Mantoo, "Vulnerability and Shame in Medicine," April 24, 2020, https://medium.com/@Uniq orndoc/vulnerability-and-shame-in-medicine-e4dc6fbba387.

39   *At least 115,000 health-care workers worldwide*: "Health and Care Worker Deaths During COVID-19," World Health Organization, October 20, 2021, https://www.who.int/news/item/20-10-2021-health-and-care-worker -deaths-during-covid-19.

3. Why Compassion, Empathy, and Respect Matter

45   *In a press release responding to her allegations*: Bill Hutchinson, "Hospital CEO's Response to Black Doctor's COVID-19 Death Prompts Backlash," *ABC News*, December 30, 2020, https://abcnews.go.com/US/hospital-ceos-response -black-doctors-covid-19-death/story?id=74971005.

46   *He told* ABC News *that his mother knew*: Hutchinson, "Hospital CEO's Response to Black Doctor's COVID-19 Death Prompts Backlash."

47   *More Black medical professionals speak up*: Aletha Maybank, Camara Phyllis Jones, Uché Blackstok, and Joia Crear-Perry, "Say Her Name: Dr. Susan Moore," *Washington Post*, December 26, 2020, https://www.washington post.com/opinions/2020/12/26/say-her-name-dr-susan-moore/.

48   *findings from an external review panel*: "Statement from IU Health CEO Dennis Murphy on External Review of Dr. Susan Moore's Care," Indiana University Heath, press release, May 12, 2021, https://iuhealth.org/for-media/press -releases/statement-from-iu-health-ceo-dennis-murphy-on-external-review -of-dr-susan-moores-care.

50   *"Empathy is*: "Priority: Teaching Empathy to Medical Students," Consult QD, Cleveland Clinic, https://consultqd.clevelandclinic.org/priority-teaching-em pathy-to-medical-students/#:~:text=%E2%80%9CEmpathy%20is%20not %20an%20option,third%2Dyear%20students%20at%20CCLCM.

50   *In one study, higher scores*: Mohammadreza Hojat, Daniel Z. Louis, Kaye Maxwell, Fred Markham, Richard Wender, and Joseph S. Gonnella, "Patient Perceptions of Physician Empathy, Satisfaction with Physician, Interpersonal Trust, and Compliance," *International Journal of Medical Education* 1 (December 14, 2010): 83–87, https://www.ncbi.nlm.nih.gov/pmc/articles/PMC 4205510/.

4. The Art and Science of Doctoring

66   *In 2021, only 36 percent of people who*: "2021 FACTS: Applicants and Matriculants Data," Association of American Medical Colleges, https://www.aamc.org/data -reports/students-residents/interactive-data/2021-facts-applicants-and-matricu lants-data.

6. Our Biased Brain

93   *we should not assume*: Martie G. Haselton, Daniel Nettle, and Damian R Murray, "The Evolution of Cognitive Bias," in *The Handbook of Evolutionary Psychology*, ed. David M. Buss (Hoboken, NJ: Wiley, 2015), 724–46, https:// doi.org/10.1002/9781119125563.evpsych241.

93   *In one study, infants were shown faces*: Naiqi G. Xiao, Paul C. Quinn, Shaoying Liu, Liezhong Ge, Olivier Pascalis, and Kang Lee, "Older but Not Younger Infants Associate Own-Race Faces with Happy Music and Other-Race Faces

with Sad Music," *Developmental Science* 21, no. 2 (February 2017), https://doi.org/10.1111/desc.12537.

93   *In another study, four-year-old boys*: Danielle R. Perszyk, Ryan F. Lei, Galen V. Bodenhausen, Jennifer A. Richeson, and Sandra R. Waxman, "Bias at the Intersection of Race and Gender: Evidence from Preschool-Aged Children," *Developmental Science* 22, no. 3 (May 2019), https://doi.org/10.1111/desc.12788.

94   *In a study published*: Andrew R. Todd, Austin Simpson, Kelsey Thiem, and Rebecca Neel, "The Generalization of Implicit Racial Bias to Young Black Boys: Automatic Stereotyping or Automatic Prejudice?" *Social Cognition* 34, no. 4 (August 2016): 306–23, https://doi.org/10.1521/soco.2016.34.4.306.

94   *According to the U.S. Department of Justice*: "Bias Policing Overview and Resource Guide," Community Relations Services, U.S. Department of Justice, https://www.justice.gov/file/1437326/download.

95   *Implicit preferences once formed*: Aiden P. Gregg, Beale Seibt, and Mahzarin R. Banaji, "Easier Done than Undone: Asymmetry in the Malleability of Implicit Preferences," *Journal of Personality and Social Psychology* 90, no. 1 (2006): 1–20, https://doi.org/10.1037/0022-3514.90.1.1.

95   *Similar findings published in 2010*: Jennifer A. Joy-Gaba and Brian A. Nosek, "The Surprisingly Limited Malleability of Implicit Racial Evaluations," *Social Psychology* 41, no. 3 (January 2010): 137–46, https://doi.org/10.1027/1864-9335/a000020.

96   *A comprehensive review published in the* American Journal of Public Health: William J. Hall, Mimi V. Chapman, Kent M. Lee, Yesenia M. Merino, Tainayah W. Thomas, B. Keith Payne, Eugenia Eng, Steven H. Day, and Tamera Coyne-Beasley, "Implicit Racial/Ethnic Bias Among Health Care Professionals and Its Influence on Health Care Outcomes: A Systematic Review," *American Journal of Public Health* 105, no. 12 (December 2015), https://doi.org/10.2105/ajph.2015.302903.

96   *In the* Journal of General Internal Medicine: Elizabeth N. Chapman, Anna Kaatz, and Molly Carnes, "Physicians and Implicit Bias: How Doctors May Unwittingly Perpetuate Health Care Disparities," *Journal of General Internal Medicine* 28 (2013): 1504–10, https://doi.org/10.1007/s11606-013-2441-1.

96   *I was puzzled*: Cristina M. Gonzalez, Mimi Y. Kim, and Paul R. Marantz, "Implicit Bias and Its Relation to Health Disparities: A Teaching Program and Survey of Medical Students," *Teaching and Learning in Medicine* 26, no. 1 (January 2014): 64–71, https://doi.org/10.1080/10401334.2013.857341.

7. The Threat from Medical Racism

118   *In urban environments, studies suggest that:* Rohan Khazanchi, Charlesnika T. Evans, and Jasmine R. Marcelin, "Racism, Not Race, Drives Inequity Across the COVID-19 Continuum," JAMA Network Open 3, no. 9 (September 25, 2020), https://jamanetwork.com/journals/jamanetworkopen/fullarticle/2770954.

119   *A study published in 2021 points out that for most cancers:* Reginald D. Tucker-Seeley, "Social Determinants of Health and Disparities in Cancer Care for Black People in the United States," *JCO Oncology Practice* 17, no. 5 (May 2021): 261–63, https://doi.org/10.1200/OP.21.00229.

120   *research on more than 172,549 healthy children*: Olubukola O. Nafiu, Christian Mpody, Stephani S. Kim, Joshua C. Uffman, and Joseph D. Tobias, "Race, Postoperative Complications, and Death in Apparently Healthy Children," *Pediatrics* 146, no. 2 (August 2020), https://doi.org/10.1542/peds.2019-4113.

120   *A 2019 study that asked subjects*: Kelly M. Hoffman, et al. "Racial Bias in Pain Assessment and Treatment Recommendations, and False Beliefs About Biological Differences Between Blacks and Whites."

123   *Asian American patients also felt them*: Ivy K. Ho and Jason Lawrence, "The Role of Social Cognition in Medical Decision Making with Asian American Patients," *Journal of Racial and Ethnic Health Disparities* 8 (October 2021): 1112–18, https://www.ncbi.nlm.nih.gov/pmc/articles/PMC7489188/.

123   *For example, nursing and medical students*: Meghan G. Bean, Elizabeth S. Focella, Rebbeca Covarrubias, Jeff Stone, Gordan B. Moskowitz, and Terry A. Badger, "Documenting Nursing and Medical Students' Stereotypes about Hispanic and American Indian Patients," *Journal of Health Disparities Research and Practice* 7, no 4 (October 2014): 14.

125   *A U.S. government–published fact sheet*: "Tips for Disaster Responders: Understanding Historical Trauma When Responding to an Event in Indian Country," Substance Abuse and Mental Health Services Administration, https://store.samhsa.gov/sites/default/files/d7/priv/sma14-4866.pdf.

128   *As the authors of* Cultural Religious Competence in Clinical Practice: Diana L. Swihart, Siva Naga S. Yarrarapu, and Romaine L. Martin, *Cultural Religious Competence in Clinical Practice* (Treasure Island, FL: StatPearls, 2022), https://www.ncbi.nlm.nih.gov/books/NBK493216/.

8. Dismissing Women, Gender Identity, and Sexual Orientation

134   *Non-Hispanic Black women*: Elizabeth A. Howell, "Reducing Disparities in Severe Maternal Morbidity and Mortality," *Clinical Obstetrics and Gynecology* 61,
no. 2 (June 2018): 387–99, https://doi.org/10.1097/GRF.0000000000000349.

135   *A 2020 report*: Laurie Zephyrin, Lisa Suennen, Pavitra Viswanathan, Jared Au-
genstein, and Deborah Bachrach, "Transforming Primary Health Care for
Women—Part 1: A Framework for Addressing Gaps and Barriers," Commonwealth Fund, July 16, 2020, https://www.commonwealthfund.org/publications
/fund-reports/2020/jul/transforming-primary-health-care-women-part-1
-framework.

137   *An estimated 5.6 percent of Americans identify*: Jeffrey M. Jones, "LGBT Identification Rises to 5.6% in Latest U.S. Estimate," Gallup, February 24, 2021,
https://news.gallup.com/poll/329708/lgbt-identification-rises-latest
-estimate.aspx.

138   *One study in Pittsburgh, Pennsylvania*: Ashley J. Simenson, Stephanie Corey,
Nina Markovic, and Suzanne Kinsky, "Disparities in Chronic Health Outcomes and Health Behaviors Between Lesbian and Heterosexual Adult
Women in Pittsburgh: A Longitudinal Study," *Journal of Women's Health* 29,
no. 8 (August 2020): 1059–67, http://doi.org/10.1089/jwh.2019.8052.

139   *Five years later*: Alex Schmider, "New U.S. Transgender Survey Has Compelling
Data About Being Trans in America: The Report of the 2015 U.S. Transgender
Survey" GLAAD, December 8, 2016, https://www.glaad.org/blog/new-us
-transgender-survey-has-compelling-data-about-being-trans-america.

142   *The CDC's social health data analysis*: "Lesbian, Gay, Bisexual, and Transgender
Health," Office of Disease Prevention and Health Promotion, https://www
.healthypeople.gov/2020/topics-objectives/topic/lesbian-gay-bisexual-and
-transgender-health.

142   *who identify as LGBT and our society*: Ibid.

143   *More than 53.7 percent of the students*: Brendan Murphy, "Women in Medical
Schools: Dig into Latest Record-Breaking Numbers," AMA, September 29, 2021,
https://www.ama-assn.org/education/medical-school-diversity/women
-medical-schools-dig-latest-record-breaking-numbers.

143   *One study discovered that if their surgeon is male*: Andrea N. Riner and Amalia
Cochran, "Surgical Outcomes Should Know No Identity—The Case for Equity
Between Patients and Surgeons," *JAMA Surgery* 157, no. 2 (February 2022): 156–
57, https://doi: 10.1001/jamasurg.2021.6367.

144   *one study suggests that burnout*: Mark Linzer and Eileen Harwood, "Gendered
Expectations: Do They Contribute to High Burnout Among Female Physi-

cians?" *Journal of General Internal Medicine* 33 (June 2018): 963–65, https://doi
.org/10.1007/s11606-018-4330-0.

9. The Perils of Ageism

146   *In fact, 82 percent of Americans*: "Everyday Ageism and Health," National Poll
on Healthy Aging, University of Michigan, July 2020, https://deepblue.lib
.umich.edu/bitstream/handle/2027.42/156038/0192_NPHA-ageism
-report_FINAL-07132020.pdf?sequence=3&isAllowed=y.

146   *One of my favorite studies on aging is the Blue Zone Project*: Dan Buettner and
Sam Skemp, "Blue Zones: Lessons from the World's Longest Lived," *American
Journal of Lifestyle Medicine* 10, no. 5 (July 2016): 318–21, https:// doi:10.1177
/1559827616637066.

148   *According to the CDC*: "Minorities and Women Are at Greater Risk for
Alzheimer's Disease," Alzheimer's Disease and Healthy Aging Program,
Centers for Disease Control and Prevention, August 20, 2019, https://www
.cdc.gov/aging/publications/features/Alz-Greater-Risk.html.

148   *It is estimated that*: "Mental Health of Older Adults," World Health Organization, December 12, 2017, https://www.who.int/news-room/fact-sheets/detail
/mental-health-of-older-adults.

149   *For example, in a study of nine thousand hospitalized*: Mary Beth Hamel, Joan
M. Teno, Lee Goldman, Joanne Lynn, Roger B. Davis, Anthony N. Galanos,
Norman A. Desbiens, Alfred F. Connors, Jr., Neil S. Wenger, and Russell S.
Phillips, "Patient Age and Decisions to Withhold Life-Sustaining Treatments
from Seriously Ill, Hospitalized Adults," *Annals of Internal Medicine* 130, no. 2
(January 19, 1999): 116–25, https://pubmed.ncbi.nlm.nih.gov/10068357/.

152   *study of French oncologists' treatment decisions*: Christel Protière, Patrice Viens,
Frédérique Rousseau, and Jean Paul Moatti, "Prescribers' Attitudes Toward
Elderly Breast Cancer Patients. Discrimination or Empathy?" *Critical Reviews
in Oncology/Hematology* 75, no. 2 (August 2010): 138–50, https://doi.org/10.1016
/j.critrevonc.2009.09.007.

152   *The World Health Organization (WHO)*: "Mental Health of Older Adults."

155   *2020 AARP survey*: Deborah Schoch, "1 in 5 Americans Now Provide Unpaid
Family Care: New AARP Research Finds Caregivers Now Top 53 Million in
U.S.," AARP, June 18, 2020, https://www.aarp.org/caregiving/basics/info
-2020/unpaid-family-caregivers-report.html.

157   *"Undervaluing older adults"*: Sharon K. Inouye, "Creating an Anti-Ageist Health-
care System to Improve Care for Our Current And Future Selves," *Nature Aging* 1
(February 2021): 150–52, https://doi.org/10.1038/s43587-020-00004-4.

10. How We Devalue People with Disabilities

162   *One in three adults with disabilities*: Lisa I. Iezzoni, "Stigma and Persons with Disabilities," in *Stigma and Prejudice: Touchstones in Understanding Diversity in Healthcare*, ed. Ranna Parekh and Ed W. Childs (Totowa, NJ: Humana Press, 2016), 3.

162   *In a survey of 714 practicing physicians nationwide*: Lisa I. Iezzoni, Sowmya R. Rao, Julie Ressalam, Dragana Bolcic-Jankovic, Nicole D. Agaronnik, Karen Donelan, Tara Lagu, and Eric G. Campbell, "Physicians' Perceptions of People with Disability and Their Health Care," *Health Affairs* 40, no. 2 (February 2021), https://www.healthaffairs.org/doi/10.1377/hlthaff.2020.01452.

165   *The National Council on Disability (NCD) issued a statement*: "NCD Chairman Statement on Death of Michael Hickson," National Council on Disability, July 2, 2020, https://ncd.gov/newsroom/2020/ncd-chairman-statement-michael-hickson-death#:~:text=Hickson%20to%20have%20a%20low,they%20rely%20on%20for%20care.

169   *"Explicit and implicit discriminatory bias within the health care professions"*: Andrés J. Gallegos "Misperceptions of People with Disabilities Lead to Low-Quality Care: How Policy Makers Can Counter the Harm and Injustice," HealthAffairs, April 1, 2021, https://www.healthaffairs.org/do/10.1377/forr front.20210325.480382.

11. Dealing with the Shame of Obesity

175   *a* New York Times *article*: Gina Kolata, "Why Do Obese Patients Get Worse Care? Many Doctors Don't See Past the Fat," *New York Times*, September 25, 2016, https://www.nytimes.com/2016/09/26/health/obese-patients-health-care.html.

177   *One national study of almost five thousand first-year medical students*: Sean M. Phelan, John F. Dovidio, Rebecca M. Puhl, Diana J. Burgess, David B. Nelson, Mark W. Yeazel, Rachel Hardeman, Sylvia Perry, and Michelle van Ryn, "Implicit and Explicit Weight Bias in a National Sample of 4732 Medical Students: The Medical Student CHANGES Study," *Obesity* 22, no. 4 (April 2014): 1201–8, https://onlinelibrary.wiley.com/doi/10.1002/oby.20687.

12. Social Determinants of Health

190   *Research has determined that improvements in education*: Steven H. Woolf, Robert E. Johnson, Robert L. Phillips, and Maike Philipsen, "Giving Everyone the Health of the Educated: An Examination of Whether Social Change Would

Save More Lives than Medical Advances," *American Journal of Public Health* 97, no. 4 (April 2007): 679–83, https://doi.org/10.2105/ajph.2005.084848.

190   *A 2014 study analyzed nitrogen dioxide*: Lara P. Clark, Dylan B. Millet, and Julian D. Marshall, "National Patterns in Environmental Injustice and Inequality: Outdoor NO$_2$ Air Pollution in the United States," *PLOS ONE* 9, no. 4 (April 2014), https://doi.org/10.1371/journal.pone.0094431.

191   *As stated by the American Public Health Association*: "Racism Is an Ongoing Public Health Crisis That Needs Our Attention Now," American Public Health Association, May 29, 2020, https://www.apha.org/news-and-media/news releases/apha-news-releases/2020/racism-is-a-public-health-crisis.

192   *According to a report by the National Women's Law Center*: "National Snapshot: Poverty Among Women & Families, 2019," National Women's Law Center, October 23, 2019, https://nwlc.org/resource/national-snapshot-poverty-among -women-families-2019/.

193   *According to the U.S. Census Bureau*: "Income, Poverty and Health Insurance Coverage in the United States: 2020," United States Census Bureau, September 14, 2021, https://www.census.gov/newsroom/press-releases/2021/income-poverty -health-insurance-coverage.html.

194   *Agency for Healthcare Research and Quality*: "2017 National Healthcare Quality and Disparities Report," Agency for Healthcare Research and Quality, reviewed July 2019, https://www.ahrq.gov/research/findings/nhqrdr/nhqdr17/index.html.

13. Science as an Invasive Health-Care Influence

201   *While many thanked her*: Kathryn Ivey, "Nurses Struggle Through a New COVID Wave with Rage and Compassion," *Scientific American*, January 11, 2022, https://www.scientificamerican.com/article/nurses-struggle-through-a-new -covid-wave-with-rage-and-compassion/.

202   *"To fully explain today's"*: Andrew Jewett, "How Americans Came to Distrust Science," *Boston Review*, December 8, 2020, https://bostonreview.net/articles /andrew-jewett-science-under-fire/.

203   *If I refuse to take the cure from my doctor*: Robert Crease, "What Is the Difference Between Science Denial, Pseudoscience, and Skepticism?" *Forbes*, April 12, 2019, https://www.forbes.com/sites/quora/2019/04/12/what-is-the-difference -between-science-denial-pseudoscience-and-skepticism/?sh=2c120da4ff4e.

203   *The science denial used to deny the existence*: Christos Makridis and Jonathan T. Rothwell, "The Real Cost of Political Polarization: Evidence from the COVID-19 Pandemic," *SSRN* (June 29, 2020), https://doi.org/10.2139/ssrn.3638373.

203   *A 10 percent increase in Fox News viewership*: Andrey Simonov, Szymon K. Sacher, Jean-Pierre H. Dubé, and Shirsho Biswas, "The Persuasive Effect of Fox News: Non-Compliance with Social Distancing during the Covid-19 Pandemic," National Bureau of Economic Research (May 2020), https://doi.org/10.3386/w27237.

203   *Republican-led states had*: Brian Neelon, Fedelis Mutiso, Noel T. Mueller, John L. Pearce, and Sara E. Benjamin-Neelon, "Associations between Governor Political Affiliation and COVID-19 Cases, Deaths, and Testing in the U.S," *American Journal of Preventive Medicine* 61, no. 1 (March 2021): 115–19, https://doi.org/10.1016/j.amepre.2021.01.034.

204   *In Gallup Polls' annual Confidence in Institutions survey*: Jeffrey M. Jones, "Democratic, Republican Confidence in Science Diverges," Gallup, July 16, 2021, https://news.gallup.com/poll/352397/democratic-republican-confidence-science-diverges.aspx.

14. Technology as an Invasive Health-Care Influence

211   *Surveys have shown that while minority patients were significantly less*: Christian Johnson, Chelsea Richwine, and Vaishali Patel, "Individuals' Access and Use of Patient Portals and Smartphone Health Apps, 2020," Office of the National Coordinator for Health Information Technology, ONC Data Brief No. 57, September 2021, https://www.healthit.gov/sites/default/files/page/2021-09/HINTS_2020_Consumer_Data_Brief.pdf.

15. Pharma and Research as an Invasive Health-Care Influence

219   *Women experience adverse drug reactions*: Elizabeth Cooney, "Females Are Still Routinely Left Out of Biomedical Research—and Ignored in Analyses of Data," STAT, June 9, 2020, https://www.statnews.com/2020/06/09/females-are-still-routinely-left-out-of-biomedical-research-and-ignored-in-analyses-of-data/.

221   *Researchers have found that Black patients*: Bassel Nazha, Manoj Mishra, Rebecca Pentz, and Taofeek K. Owonikoko, "Enrollment of Racial Minorities in Clinical Trials: Old Problem Assumes New Urgency in the Age of Immunotherapy," *American Society of Clinical Oncology Educational Book* 39 (May 2019): 3–10, https://doi.org/10.1200/EDBK_100021.

221   *Yet even in the NIH, funding proposal*: Anna Volerman, Vineet M. Arora, John F. Cursio, Helen Wei, and Valerie G. Press, "Representation of Women on Na-

tional Institutes of Health Study Sections," *JAMA Network Open* 4, no. 2 (February 2021), https://doi.org/10.1001/jamanetworkopen.2020.37346.

16. Payment Systems as an Invasive Health-Care Influence

232   *According to the American Medical Association*: Devorah Goldman, "The Doctor's Office Becomes an Assembly Line," *Wall Street Journal*, December 29, 2021, https://www.wsj.com/articles/doctors-office-becomes-an-assembly-line-family-private-physician-hospital-medicare-reimbursement-ehr-medical-drug-price-cost-11640791761.

Index